Diabetes Cooking **101**

Cover photo © Brave New Pictures.

Food Stylist: Mary Valentin

Photos on the following pages from Shutterstock: 4, 10, 13, 16, 17, 18, 19, 20, 24, 36, 46, 56, 70, 84, 96, 102, 114, 124.

Photos on the following pages from Brave New Pictures: 29, 43, 53, 61, 67, 75, 79, 93, 109, 119, 129, 143.

Printed in China.

Library of Congress Cataloging-in-Publication Data

Diabetes cooking 101 : master diabetes cooking with 101 great recipes / edited by Perrin Davis.
    p. cm.
Includes index.
ISBN-13: 978-1-57284-127-7 (flexibound)
ISBN-10: 1-57284-127-3 (flexibound)
ISBN-13: 978-1-57284-695-1 (ebook)
ISBN-10: 1-57284-695-X (ebook)
1. Diabetes--Diet therapy--Recipes. 2. Cookbooks. I. Davis, Perrin, 1969-
  RC662.D5215 2011
641.56314--dc23

                          2011039678

16 15 14 13 12   10 9 8 7 6 5 4 3 2 1

Surrey Books is an imprint of Agate Publishing, Inc.

Agate and Surrey books are available in bulk at discount prices. For more information, go to

agatepublishing.com.

Diabetes Cooking **101**

MASTER DIABETES COOKING WITH 101 GREAT RECIPES

EDITED BY Perrin Davis

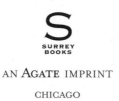

S

SURREY
BOOKS

AN AGATE IMPRINT

CHICAGO

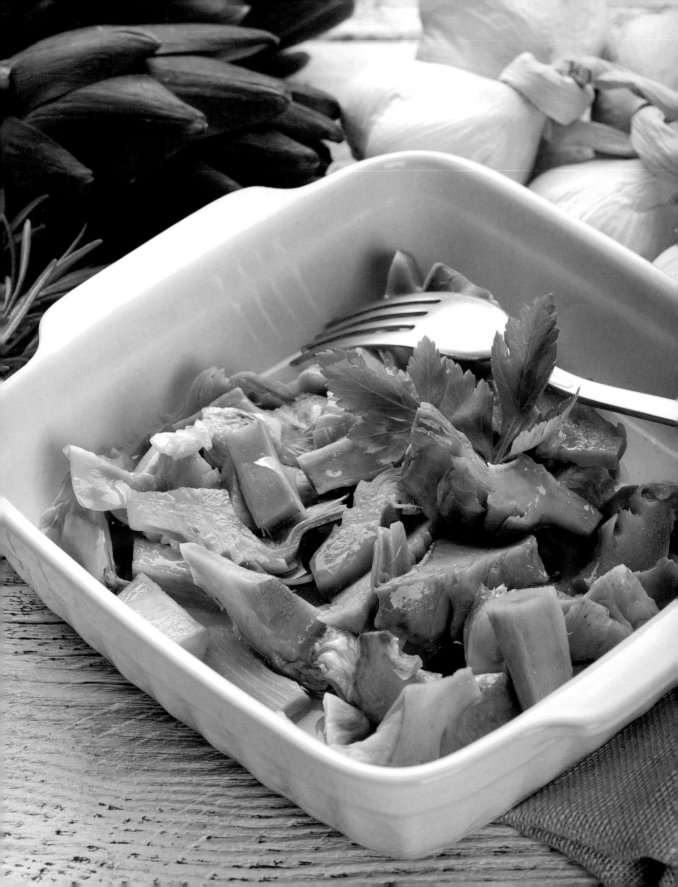

CONTENTS

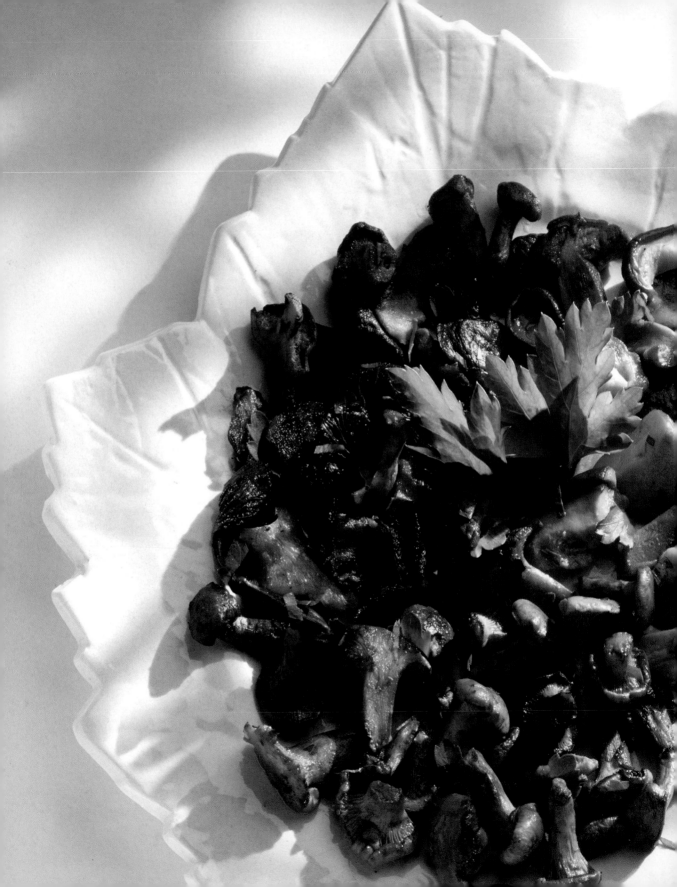

INTRODUCTION

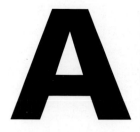gate Surrey Books wants to help everyone, but especially kitchen beginners, learn how to explore different kinds of food and cooking. We are proud to introduce the *101* series, which aims to provide rewarding, successful, and fun cooking experiences for everyone, from novices to more experienced cooks. *Diabetes Cooking 101: Master Diabetes Cooking with 101 Great Recipes* is one of the first books in this series, and it offers readers not only delicious recipes but also useful information about shopping for equipment, ingredients, kitchen essentials, and seasonings. Getting started with diabetes cooking can be intimidating, but we'll demystify the process for you. So whether you or someone you love has just recently been diagnosed with diabetes, or if you have been dealing with the disease for some time, *Diabetes Cooking 101* is a great place to start.

Most of the recipes in the *101* series books come from a wide range of Agate Surrey authors and editors. Contributors to *Diabetes Cooking 101* include Sue Spitler, editor of the "1,001" series that includes titles like *1,001 Delicious Recipes for People with Diabetes* and *1,001 Delicious Desserts for People with Diabetes*, and Barbara Grunes, author of *Diabetes Snacks, Treats, and Easy Eats: 130 Recipes You'll Make Again and Again* and *Diabetes Snacks, Treats, and Easy Eats for Kids: 130 Recipes for the Foods Kids Really Like to Eat*.

Diabetes Cooking 101 recipes were selected to provide a starting point for anyone beginning their diabetes cooking journey. The collection includes a variety of cuisines (Italian, Mexican, Spanish, Asian, and Greek, to name a few). Most of the recipes are simple, although a handful of them are more advanced; you'll find that all are easy to follow.

A TASTE OF WHAT YOU'LL FIND IN THIS BOOK

This book contains lots of fantastic main-dish options in the Beef, Chicken, and Seafood Entrées chapters. Don't miss great dinner-party options like Steak au Poivre, Shish Kebabs, Flank

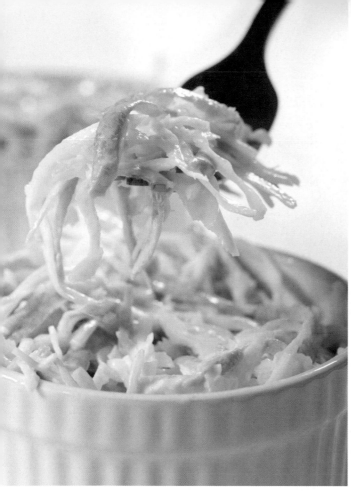

Steak on Salad Greens, and Chicken Cordon Bleu, as well as delicious family pleasers like Chicken and Cheese Rellenos and Soft Tacos. Scallops with Asparagus and Crab Cakes will put smiles on everyone's face, and Halibut with Sour Cream and Poblano Sauce is a big favorite in our house.

In the Side Dishes chapter, check out delicious dishes like Mushrooms with Sour Cream, Eggplant and Vegetable Sauté, Broccoli Rabe Sautéed with Garlic, and Asparagus with Lemon-Wine Sauce.

Looking for a delightful bread option to serve with dinner? Try the Roasted Red Pepper Bread or the Cheddar Biscuits! Cheesecake Cupcakes, Biscotti, and Chocolate Chip Cookies are just a few of the tasty, low-sugar, and low-carbohydrate offerings in the Desserts chapter. Need to delight a more sophisticated palate? Look no further than our Strawberry Cream Pie on page 128.

But before you get started cooking some of these great recipes, make sure you're up to speed on some diabetes cooking basics, and that your kitchen and pantry are ready to go!

DIABETES COOKING BASICS

Have you or someone you love been diagnosed with diabetes; prediabetes, a condition that involves blood glucose levels that are higher than normal but not high enough to be considered diabetic level; or metabolic syndrome, a condition in which one's body does not use insulin effectively? If so, it's likely that the doctor advised a change in diet. A sensible diet for a diabetic or pre-diabetic person is low in fat, low in sugar, low in calories, low in carbohydrates, rich in monounsaturated fats, and includes a wide variety of different types of food. That may sound very daunting to you, but this book proves that you can follow all those guidelines and still enjoy delicious foods.

When planning meals, watch your carbohydrate intake carefully. You should have approximately the same quantity of carbohydrates at each meal (usually no more than 30 to 45 grams per meal). The American Diabetes Association suggests that you focus on portion sizes at each meal, eating small portions of meats or meat substitutes and starchy foods (like whole-grain pasta and breads, brown rice, or sweet potatoes) and large portions of nonstarchy vegetables, such as spinach, green beans, cucumbers, mushrooms, beets, broccoli, cabbage, or cauliflower. In the pages of this book, you'll find a number of terrific recipes for each of these delicious options.

Of course, it is always critical to follow the guidance of your doctor regarding any specific directions you are given about diet. This book is not meant to supply medical advice or diet guidelines, but instead to give you a general sense of how to prepare meals that follow the basic eating guidelines observed by many people who are coping with diabetes.

KITCHEN EQUIPMENT BASICS

If you are a new cook, or it's been a while since you've spent time in the kitchen, here is some helpful information that will make it easy to jump into *Diabetes Cooking 101* recipes. The following is not necessarily diabetes-cooking specific, but if you have the following equipment, you will be prepared to make almost any recipe in this book.

Appliances

We're sure you know this already, but your kitchen should include the following standard set of appliances.

Pretty Much Mandatory

- Refrigerator/freezer (set to about 34°F to 38°F [1°C to 3°C], or as cold as you can get it without freezing vegetables or drinks)

- Freezer (if yours is not frost-free, you'll periodically need to unplug it to defrost your snow-filled box)

- Stove/oven (make sure to keep the oven very clean, as burnt foods and other odors can affect the taste of your food)

- Microwave (again, make sure it's clean and ready for use), because it's great for defrosting

- Blender (and not just for beverages and soups—you can use it in place of a food processor or an immersion blender in some instances)

- Hand mixer (well, you can always stir by hand, but sometimes, the hand mixer is indispensable)

Optional

- Food processor
- Immersion blender
- Stand mixer
- Slow cooker

Pots and Pans

The following are useful basic equipment for any kitchen.

- Stockpot (8 to 10 quarts [7.6 to 9.5 L])
- Dutch oven (5 to 6 quarts [4.7 to 5.7 L])
- Pancake griddle
- Large stockpot with lid (6 to 8 quarts [5.7 to 7.6 L])

- Large skillet with lid (10 to 12 inches in diameter [25 to 30 cm])

- Medium skillet with lid (7 to 8 inches in diameter [17.5 to 20 cm])

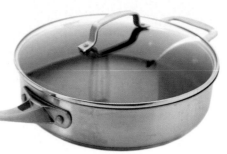

- Medium or large saucepan with lid (2 or 3 quarts [1.9 to 2.8 L])

- Small saucepan with lid (1 quart [.95 L])

- Glass casserole dish (2 quarts [1.9 L])

- Square cake pan (8 or 9 inches [20 to 22.5 cm])

- Rectangular cake pan (13 by 9 inches [32.5 by 22.5 cm])

- 2 loaf pans (8 inches [20 cm] long)

- Jelly-roll pan

- Muffin pan (12 muffins)

- Pie pan (9 inches in diameter [22.5 cm])

- 2 baking sheets

General Utensils

These are recommended basics for any kitchen.

- Knives: Chef's knife, serrated knife, and paring knife

- Measuring cups for both dry and liquid measures

- Measuring spoons

- Mixing bowls (two or three, ranging from 1 or 2 quarts to 5 or 6 quarts [.95 or 1.9 L to 4.7 or 5.7 L])

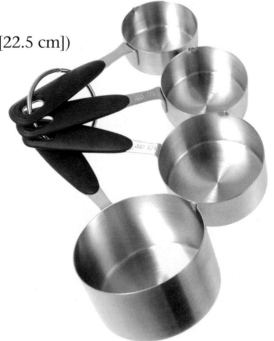

- Wooden spoons, slotted spoon, rubber or silicone spatula, ladle, whisk, tongs, and a large metal "flipper" for hamburgers and similar foods

- Colander

- Cheese grater

- Citrus zester

- Salt and pepper mills

- Kitchen scissors

- Vegetable peeler

- Can opener

- Cooling rack

- Kitchen timer

- Cutting boards—at least two, so you have one for vegetables and cooked foods and one for raw meats

- Pot holders

- Kitchen towels

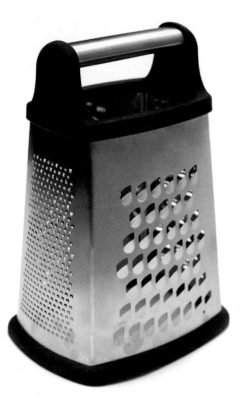

Storage and Paper Supplies

Either in a handy drawer or on a shelf, make sure you have all of these items within easy reach.

- Plastic or glass storage containers (5 to 10, varying sizes)

- Aluminum foil

- Plastic wrap

- Parchment paper

- Small baggies

- Large baggies

- Muffin cup liners

BASIC INGREDIENTS LIST FOR DIABETES COOKING

This section includes the basics that you should have on hand, but this is by no means a comprehensive list for every recipe in this book. If you have these ingredients as a starting point, however, you'll be in great shape to tackle almost any of the *Diabetes Cooking 101* recipes!

Seasonings and Flavorings

- Bay leaves
- Cayenne pepper
- Chili powder
- Ground cumin
- Dry mustard
- Garlic powder
- Ground cinnamon
- Ground ginger
- Ground nutmeg
- Red pepper flakes
- Rosemary
- Italian seasoning
- Oregano
- Paprika
- Kosher salt
- Vanilla extract
- White pepper
- Freshly ground black pepper
- Beef, chicken, and vegetable bouillon cubes or base (just add water to them to make instant stock)

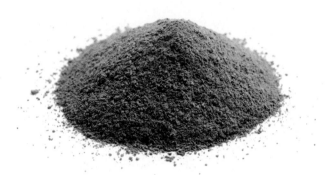
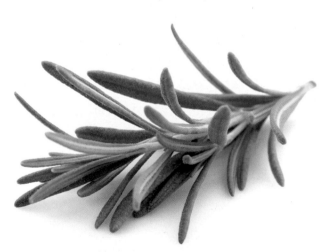

Condiments

- Apple cider vinegar
- Balsamic vinegar
- Honey
- Hot pepper sauce
- Ketchup
- Mustard
- Olive oil
- Red wine vinegar
- Rice vinegar
- Soy sauce
- Vegetable oil
- White wine vinegar
- Worcestershire sauce

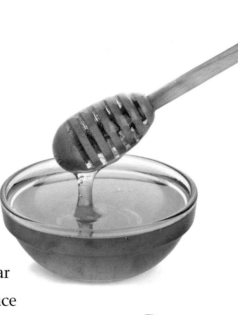

Baking

- Cornstarch
- Baking powder
- Baking soda
- Margarine
- Vegetable shortening
- Fat-free milk
- Stevia-based sweetener (see photo at right)
- Maple syrup
- Molasses
- Equal® for Recipes or Equal® sweetener in individual packets

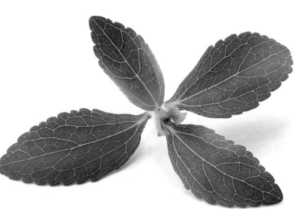

- Granulated sugar
- Light brown sugar
- Unbleached all-purpose flour
- Unbleached whole wheat flour
- Unbleached white spelt flour
- Fat-free, nondairy whipped topping
- Dutch process cocoa powder
- Fresh large eggs or egg substitute

General

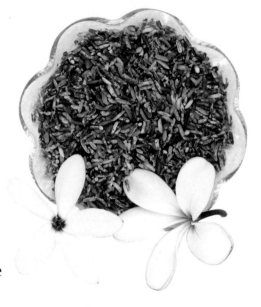

- Brown rice
- Garlic
- Whole wheat pasta
- Onions
- Canned tomatoes
- Lentils
- Raisins
- Tomato sauce
- Beef, chicken, and vegetable broth

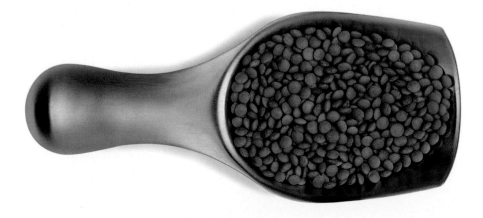

COMMON COOKING TERMS

You probably are quite familiar with most of these terms. If this is your first time cooking or it's been a while since you've been in the kitchen, here is a quick refresher:

- **Brown:** To cook a meat at a high temperature for a very brief period of time in order to seal in the juices and add lots of flavor. You'll see this in a lot of this book's recipes, because it's a tremendous flavor booster. Browning should take no more than 2 or 3 minutes on each side and is done before thoroughly cooking the meat. It may be tempting to skip this step, but please don't...it's really worth the few minutes in terms of the flavor and texture of the meat once your recipe is complete.

- **Bake:** To cook food with dry heat, usually in the oven at a specified temperature.

- **Boil:** To cook food in boiling water (212°F [100°C]) on the stovetop.

- **Blanch:** A technique that involves immersing food in boiling water for a brief period of time and then immediately transferring into an ice bath in order to stop the cooking process. Blanching is an excellent technique for quickly cooking tender vegetables, as it helps them retain their firmness, crispness, and color.

- **Braise:** This technique is a combination of browning the surface of meat, which means to cook at a high temperature for a short amount of time, followed by cooking at a lower temperature in a covered pot with liquid for a longer period of time.

- **Broil:** To cook over a high heat at a specified distance from the heat source, usually in the oven or in the "broiler" part of the oven.

- **Deep fry:** To cook food by immersing it in preheated oil.

- **Grill:** To cook over an open flame on a metal framework, grid, or other cooking surface.

- **Roast:** To cook meat in an oven in an uncovered dish, usually resulting in a well-browned surface that seals in juices and flavors.

- **Sauté:** To cook food over a medium-high or high heat in a skillet or sauté pan in a small amount of oil, water, stock, or other liquid.

- **Steam:** To cook food with steam, usually in a steamer rack or basket positioned over (but not immersed in) a pan containing a small amount of water.

- **Stir-fry:** To cook over high heat with a small amount of oil; usually requires regular stirring as food is cooking. It can be used for several kinds of dishes and is often associated with Asian fare.

GENERAL COOKING TIPS

No matter what you're cooking or how many people you're serving, a few universal rules of the kitchen will make your life easier. The following is a list of our recommendations for the novice cook. These great habits will ensure fewer mistakes, less stress, and ultimately more delicious food.

- **Read every recipe from beginning to end, at least twice, before you start cooking.** This will help to ensure that you understand how it should be made and what you need to make it.

- **Set up your ingredients, pots, pans, and utensils before you begin to prepare the recipes.** We never start a recipe until we have every ingredient on the counter in front of us. (If possible, we also premeasure all the ingredients and have them ready to add, because there's nothing worse than accidentally dumping half a box of kosher salt into an almost-finished recipe.) If you know you'll need a greased pan in step 4, grease it and set it aside before you even get started.

- **Keep a grocery list and a pen attached to the refrigerator.** If you go to the grocery store without a specific list of what you need, you're likely to forget at least a few items.

- **Clean up as you go.** If you take the time to clean your dishes as you're cooking, you'll find that you will have more space to work in and less to do after the meal is done.

- **Time the meal.** It can be complicated to cook multiple recipes at once and make sure that everything ends up finishing at roughly the same time. Make sure you allow for enough time for everything to get done, and for recipes to be cooked simultaneously.

- **Be careful.** It sounds silly, but never forget that you're working with high-temperature appliances and cookware and sharp utensils! Use proper precaution when lifting lids, turning pans, and straining vegetables.

- **Have fun!** We hope you enjoy learning how to cook these recipes and sharing them with others.

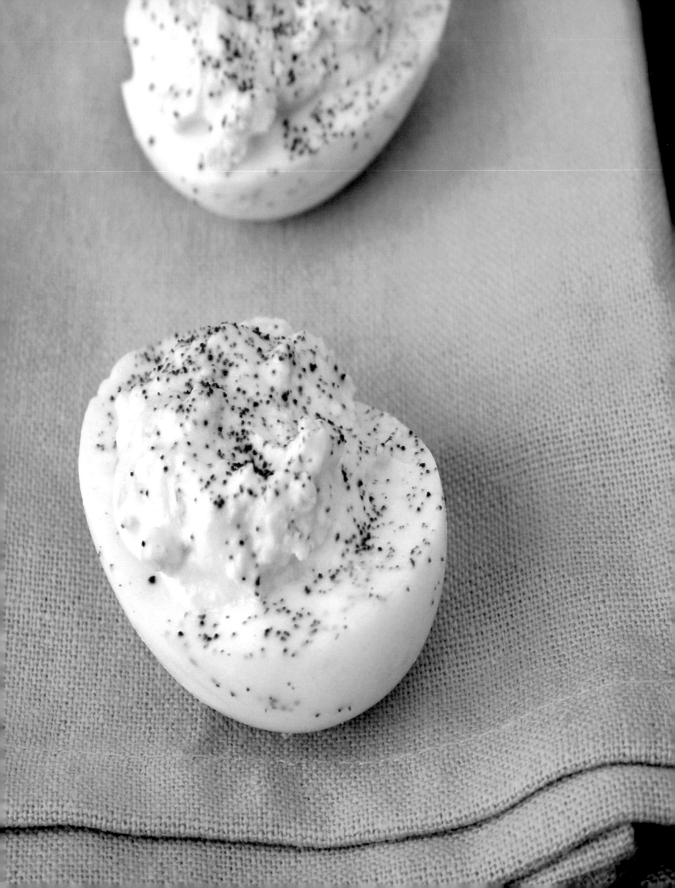

APPETIZERS AND DIPS

DEVILED EGGS

Using reduced-fat cottage cheese and nonfat salad dressing instead of traditional mayonnaise means deviled eggs can stay on your menu.

12 EGG HALVES (1 EGG HALF PER SERVING)

> 6 large eggs
> ¼ cup (59 mL) reduced-fat or fat-free cottage cheese
> 3 tablespoons (45 mL) nonfat ranch-style dressing
> 1 teaspoon (5 mL) prepared mustard
> 2 tablespoons (30 mL) finely chopped green bell pepper

1. Place the eggs in a saucepan and cover with water. Bring to boiling over medium heat. Remove saucepan from heat. Let eggs stand in pan, covered, for 20 minutes. Drain. Cool eggs and peel.

2. Slice eggs lengthwise and remove the yolks. Arrange the whites, cut side up, on a plate and cover with plastic wrap until ready to fill.

3. Combine the cottage cheese, dressing, mustard, and yolks. Mash with a fork until smooth. Mix in the bell pepper. Spoon the filling into the egg whites.

4. Cover and keep cold until ready to serve.

Serving Suggestion: Add 2 tablespoons (30 mL) of chopped fresh parsley or dill or ½ teaspoon (2.5 mL) curry powder to the filling for extra flavor.

Per Serving: Calories: 48; % calories from fat: 50; Fat (g): 2.6; Saturated fat (g): 0.8; Cholesterol (mg): 106.4; Sodium (mg): 99; Protein (g): 3.7; Carbohydrate (g): 1.9 Exchanges: Milk: 0.0; Vegetable: 0.0; Fruit: 0.0; Bread: 0.0; Meat: 0.5; Fat: 0.5

MUSHROOM BRUSCHETTA

Use any desired wild mushrooms and make this filling up to 2 days in advance.

12 SERVINGS (1 EACH)

½ cup (75 g) chopped red bell pepper
2 each: thinly sliced green onions, minced garlic cloves
2 cups (150 g) chopped wild mushrooms (portobello, shiitake, oyster, enoki, etc.)
1½ teaspoons (7.5 mL) dried basil leaves
2 tablespoons (30 mL) grated fat-free Parmesan cheese
Few drops balsamic vinegar
Salt and pepper, to taste
French bread, sliced thinly and toasted
¼ cup (59 mL) (2 ounces [56 g]) shredded reduced-fat mozzarella cheese

1. Sauté the bell pepper, green onions, and garlic 2 to 3 minutes in a lightly greased skillet. Add the mushrooms and basil and cook, covered, over medium heat until wilted, about 5 minutes. Uncover and cook until liquid is gone, 8 to 10 minutes. Stir in Parmesan cheese; season to taste with balsamic vinegar, salt, and pepper.

2. Spoon mushroom mixture onto French bread slices and sprinkle with mozzarella cheese; broil 6 inches from heat source until cheese is melted, 1 to 2 minutes.

Per Serving: Calories: 92; % of calories from fat: 17; Fat (g): 1.7; Saturated fat (g): 0.7; Cholesterol (mg): 2.5; Sodium (mg): 194; Protein (g): 4.4; Carbohydrate (g): 14.6 Exchanges: Milk: 0.0; Vegetable: 0.5; Fruit: 0.0; Bread: 1.0; Meat: 0.5; Fat: 0.0

BAKED SPINACH BALLS >

Often laden with butter, these savory treats are rich in flavor. Our version is much lower in fat.

> 2 cups (120 g) herb-seasoned bread stuffing cubes
> ¼ cup each: grated fat-free Parmesan cheese (23 g),
>   chopped green onions (25 g)
> 2 cloves garlic, minced
> ⅛ teaspoon (.625 mL) ground nutmeg
> 1 package (10 ounces [280 g]) frozen chopped spinach,
>   thawed, well drained
> ¼–⅓ cup (59–79 mL) reduced-sodium vegetable broth
> 2 tablespoons (30 mL) margarine or butter, melted
> Salt and pepper, to taste
> 1 egg, lightly beaten

1. Combine the stuffing cubes, Parmesan cheese, onions, garlic, and nutmeg in medium bowl. Mix in the spinach, broth, and margarine; season to taste with salt and pepper. Mix in egg. Shape mixture into 24 balls.

2. Bake at 350°F (180°C) on a greased jelly-roll pan until spinach balls are browned, about 15 minutes.

Per Serving: Calories: 86; % of calories from fat: 24; Fat (g): 2.4; Saturated fat (g): 0.4; Cholesterol (mg): 0; Sodium (mg): 271; Protein (g): 4.2; Carbohydrate (g): 13
Exchanges: Milk: 0.0; Vegetable: 1.0; Fruit: 0.0; Bread: 0.5; Meat: 0.0; Fat: 0.5

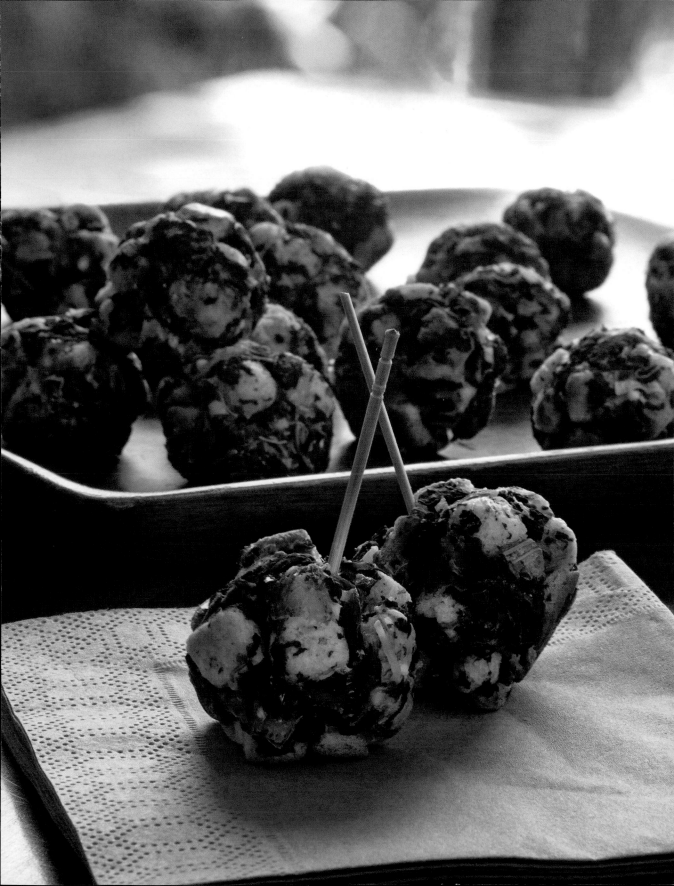

TWO-BEAN SPREAD

2 CUPS, OR 8 (¼-CUP [59-ML]) SERVINGS

  2 cloves garlic, minced
  1 can (15 ounces [425 g]) cannellini beans, rinsed, drained (see note)
  1 cup (164 g) cooked chickpeas (garbanzo beans), rinsed, drained
  3 tablespoons (45 mL) orange juice
  2 tablespoons (30 mL) extra-virgin olive oil
  1 tablespoon (15 mL) fresh lemon juice
  ⅛ teaspoon (.625 mL) pepper
  ¼ teaspoon (1.25 mL) dried basil
  Salt, to taste

1. Process the garlic, beans, chickpeas, orange juice, oil, lemon juice, pepper, and basil until smooth in a food processor, or mash together in a bowl with a potato masher. Season to taste with salt.

2. Spoon mixture into a serving bowl and garnish with parsley sprig or paprika, if desired.

Note: Cannellini beans are large white Italian kidney beans. Other white beans, such as Great Northern, can be substituted. To lower sodium in recipes, use reduced-sodium canned beans or cook your beans from scratch without salt.

Per Serving: Calories: 111; % calories from fat: 32; Fat (g): 3.9; Saturated fat (g): 0.5; Cholesterol (mg): 0; Sodium (mg): 200; Protein (g): 3.6; Carbohydrate (g): 15.2 Exchanges: Milk: 0.0; Vegetable: 0.0; Fruit: 0.0; Bread: 1.0; Meat: 0.0; Fat: 1.0

EGGPLANT DIP

Serve this dip with warm whole wheat pita halves and cut-up vegetables for dipping.

3 CUPS, OR 6 (½-CUP [59-ML]) SERVINGS

1 large purple eggplant
1 can (14½ ounces [411 g]) diced tomatoes, drained
½ cup each: chopped onion (75 g), parsley (30 g)
2 tablespoons (30 mL) red wine vinegar
1 tablespoon (15 mL) olive oil
¼ teaspoon (1.25 mL) garlic powder or dried oregano
⅛ teaspoon (.625 mL) black pepper
Salt, to taste

1. Place eggplant on a baking sheet. Bake at 375°F (190°C) 1 hour, turning occasionally, or until fork tender.

2. Remove the eggplant from the oven and cool on baking sheet. Cut lengthwise and scoop out pulp into mixing bowl. Discard skin. Mash pulp with a fork.

3. Stir in tomato, onion, parsley, vinegar, oil, garlic powder, and pepper. Season to taste with salt. Cover and refrigerate 1 hour. Stir dip before serving.

Per Serving: Calories: 65; % calories from fat: 33; Fat (g): 2.5; Saturated fat (g): 0.3; Cholesterol (mg): 0; Sodium (mg): 114; Protein (g): 1.8; Carbohydrate (g): 9.4
Exchanges: Milk: 0.0; Vegetable: 2.0; Fruit: 0.0; Bread: 0.0; Meat: 0.0; Fat: 0.5

ROASTED ZUCCHINI AND GARLIC SPREAD

A great recipe for summer, when garden zucchini are in generous supply.

12 SERVINGS (ABOUT 2 TABLESPOONS [30 ML] EACH)

1¼ pounds (568 g) zucchini, sliced (1 inch [2.5 cm])
1 small onion, cut into wedges
2 garlic cloves, peeled
⅓ cup (79 mL) fat-free plain yogurt
2 tablespoons (30 mL) chopped parsley
Lemon juice, to taste
Salt and cayenne pepper, to taste
Dippers: Assorted vegetables and crackers

1. Arrange the zucchini, onion, and garlic in single layer on a greased, foil-lined pan. Bake at 425°F (220°C) until vegetables are very tender, about 15 to 20 minutes for garlic, 25 to 30 minutes for zucchini and onion. Cool.

2. Process the vegetables in food processor until coarsely chopped. Stir in yogurt and parsley; season to taste with lemon juice, salt, and cayenne pepper. Serve with dippers (not included in nutritional data).

Per Serving: Calories: 16; % of calories from fat: 6; Fat (g): 0.1; Saturated fat (g): 0.0; Cholesterol (mg): 0.1; Sodium (mg): 11; Protein (g): 1.1; Carbohydrate (g): 3.2
Exchanges: Milk: 0.0; Vegetable: 0.5; Fruit: 0.0; Bread: 0.0; Meat: 0.0; Fat: 0.0

CALIFORNIA WRAPS

Tortillas and wraps come in a variety of flavors, including sun-dried tomato, spinach, and whole wheat. Experiment with flavors to find out what you like best. For extra flavor add dried oregano and alfalfa sprouts to the wrap.

20 SLICES (1 SLICE PER SERVING)

> 1 cup (236 mL) reduced-fat ricotta cheese
> 2 (11-inch [27.5-cm]) whole wheat flour tortillas or spinach wraps
> 1 large tomato, thinly sliced
> 2 cups (60 g) torn spinach or lettuce leaves
> 1 cup (150 g) chopped onion
> 4 ounces (112 g) thinly sliced roasted turkey breast

1. Spread ½ cup (118 mL) of cheese evenly over each tortilla to within ¼ inch (.5 cm) of the edge. Starting 1 inch (2.5 cm) from the bottom edge, layer half the tomato, spinach, onion, and turkey over the cheese onto each tortilla.

2. Starting from the bottom, roll up the wraps jelly-roll style. Wrap tightly in plastic wrap and refrigerate for 1 hour.

3. To serve, remove the plastic wrap and cut each wrap diagonally into 1-inch slices.

Per Serving: Calories: 31; % calories from fat: 13; Fat (g): 0.5; Saturated fat (g): 0.2; Cholesterol (mg): 6.9; Sodium (mg): 45; Protein (g): 4; Carbohydrate (g): 2.7 Exchanges: Milk: 0.0; Vegetable: 0.0; Fruit: 0.0; Bread: 0.0; Meat: 0.5; Fat: 0.0

MUSHROOMS STUFFED WITH ORZO

Enjoy flavor accents of tangy goat cheese and a trio of fresh herbs. This recipe comes from 1,001 Delicious Recipes for People with Diabetes by Sue Spitler.

4 SERVINGS (3 MUSHROOMS EACH)

12 large mushrooms, stems removed and chopped

1 tablespoon (15 mL) each: finely chopped shallot, garlic, fresh basil leaves

2 teaspoons (10 mL) finely chopped fresh or ½ teaspoon (2.5 mL) dried oregano leaves

½ teaspoon (2.5 mL) finely chopped fresh or ⅛ teaspoon (.625 mL) dried thyme leaves

¼ cup (59 mL) (2 ounces [56 g]) orzo, cooked

1 tablespoon goat cheese or reduced-fat cream cheese

1. Sauté the chopped mushroom stems, shallot, garlic and herbs in a lightly greased medium skillet until tender, about 6 minutes. Stir in orzo and goat cheese.

2. Spoon the filling into mushroom caps and place in 13 × 9-inch (33 cm × 23-cm) baking pan. Bake at 350°F (180°C) covered with foil, until the mushrooms are tender, about 15 minutes.

Per Serving: Calories: 86; % of calories from fat: 24; Fat (g): 2.6; Saturated fat (g): 0.6; Cholesterol (mg): 3.4; Sodium (mg): 18; Protein (g): 5.3; Carbohydrate (g): 13 Exchanges: Milk: 0.0; Vegetable: 1.0; Fruit: 0.0; Bread: 0.5; Meat: 0.0; Fat: 0.5

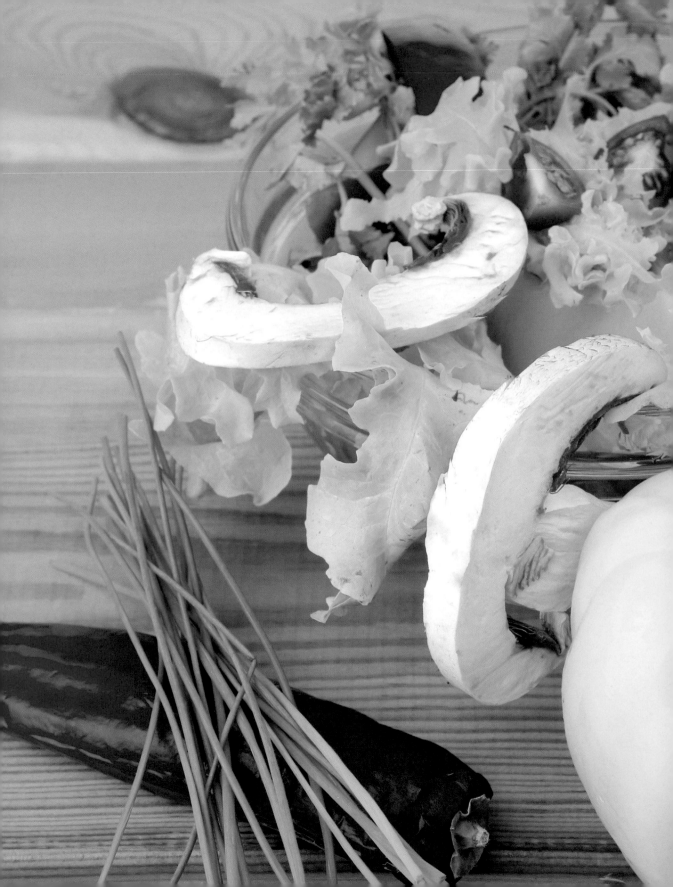

SALADS

10-LAYER SALAD

Make this salad as many layers as you want! Add a layer of cubed chicken breast or lean smoked ham for an entrée salad, using 3 ounces of cooked meat per person.

8 SERVINGS

2 cups (72 g) thinly sliced romaine lettuce
1 cup each: sliced red cabbage (90 g), mushrooms (75 g), carrots (128 g), green bell pepper (150 g), halved cherry tomatoes (160 g), small broccoli or cauliflower florets (150 g)
½ cup each: sliced cucumber (130 g), red onion (150 g)
Herbed Sour Cream Dressing (recipe follows)
Finely chopped parsley, as garnish

1. Arrange the lettuce in bottom of 1½-quart (1.5 L) glass bowl; arrange remaining vegetables in layers over lettuce. Spread Herbed Sour Cream Dressing over top of salad and sprinkle with parsley.

2. Refrigerate, loosely covered, 8 hours or overnight. Toss before serving.

HERBED SOUR CREAM DRESSING

ABOUT 1½ CUPS (354 ML)

¾ cup (177 mL) each: fat-free mayonnaise and sour cream
2–3 cloves garlic, minced
½ teaspoon (2.5 mL) each: dried basil and tarragon leaves
¼ teaspoon (1.25 mL) each: salt, pepper

1. Mix all ingredients.

Per Serving: Calories: 68; % of calories from fat: 4; Fat (g): 0.4; Saturated fat (g): 0.1; Cholesterol (mg): 0; Sodium (mg): 380; Protein (g): 3.3; Carbohydrate (g): 14.8
Exchanges: Milk: 0.0; Vegetable: 1.5; Fruit: 0.0; Bread: 0.0; Meat: 0.0; Fat: 0.0

GREEK SALAD

Pay a visit to the salad bar in your favorite supermarket. It is a convenient way to buy the "bits and pieces" and the vegetables you need.

8 (1½-CUP [354-ML]) SERVINGS

> 10 cups torn romaine lettuce
> 1 cup each: chopped fresh tomatoes (160 g), sliced red bell pepper (150 g) and cucumber (130 g)
> ¼ cup each: sliced red onions (38 g), cubed feta cheese (38 g)
> ½ cup (118 mL) low-fat Greek-style salad dressing

1. Toss together the lettuce, tomatoes, bell pepper, cucumber, onions, and cheese. Add dressing and toss again.

Per Serving: Calories: 55; % calories from fat: 50; Fat (g): 3.5; Saturated fat (g): 0.4; Cholesterol (mg): 0.8; Sodium (mg): 140; Protein (g): 1.7; Carbohydrate (g): 6.1
Exchanges: Milk: 0.0; Vegetable: 1.0; Fruit: 0.0; Bread: 0.0; Meat: 0.0; Fat: 1.0

CACTUS SALAD

The tender cactus paddles called "nopales" are readily available in large supermarkets today. Be sure all the thorns have been removed; if not, they can be pulled out easily with tweezers.

6 SERVINGS

2 quarts (1.9 L) water

1½ pounds (680 g) cactus paddles, cut into ½-inch (13-mm) pieces

1 tablespoon (15 mL) salt

¼ teaspoon (1.25 mL) baking soda

1½ cups (240 g) halved cherry tomatoes

½ cup (75 g) thinly sliced red onion

Lime Dressing (recipe follows)

1. Heat water to boiling in large saucepan; add the cactus, salt, and baking soda. Reduce heat and simmer, uncovered, until cactus is crisp-tender, about 20 minutes. Rinse in cold water; drain.

2. Place the cactus, tomatoes, and onion in salad bowl. Add Lime Dressing and toss.

LIME DRESSING

ABOUT ¼ CUP (59 ML)

2 tablespoons (30 mL) lime juice

1–2 tablespoons (15–30 mL) olive or canola oil

1 tablespoon (15 mL) water

2 teaspoons (10 mL) sugar

1 teaspoon (5 mL) cider vinegar

½ teaspoon (2.5 mL) dried oregano leaves

1. Combine all ingredients.

Per Serving: Calories: 78; % of calories from fat: 28; Fat (g): 2.5; Saturated fat (g): 0.3; Cholesterol (mg): 0; Sodium (mg): 131; Protein (g): 2.4; Carbohydrate (g): 12.5 Exchanges: Milk: 0.0; Vegetable: 2.0; Fruit: 0.0; Bread: 0.0; Meat: 0.0; Fat: 0.5

COLESLAW

For faster preparation and less waste, purchase packaged shredded cabbage, which can be found in the produce section of most supermarkets.

12 (¾-CUP [177-ML]) SERVINGS

> 6 cups (540 g) shredded green cabbage
> 2 cups (220 g) grated carrots
> ¾ cup (177 mL) fat-free mayonnaise
> ¼ cup (59 mL) red wine vinegar
> 3 tablespoons (50 g) sugar or spoonable sugar substitute
> ¼ teaspoon (1.25 mL) salt
> ½ teaspoon (2.5 mL) each: black pepper, dry mustard

1. Toss together the cabbage and carrots in a large bowl.

2. Whisk together the mayonnaise, vinegar, sugar, salt, black pepper, and mustard in a small bowl. Toss the dressing with the vegetables.

3. Serve immediately or cover with plastic wrap and refrigerate until serving time. Toss coleslaw again before serving.

Serving Suggestion: Substitute half of the green cabbage with shredded red cabbage. For extra flavor, add ½ cup sliced red onion and 1 tablespoon celery seeds.

Per Serving: Calories: 39; % calories from fat: 4; Fat (g): 0.2; Saturated fat (g): 0; Cholesterol (mg): 0; Sodium (mg): 181; Protein (g): 0.7; Carbohydrate (g): 8.8 Exchanges: Milk: 0.0; Vegetable: 2.0; Fruit: 0.0; Bread: 0.0; Meat: 0.0; Fat: 0.0

SPINACH AND MELON SALAD >

A colorful salad, accented with sweet Honey Dressing. This recipe comes from 1,001 Delicious Recipes for People with Diabetes *by Sue Spitler.*

8 SERVINGS

> 8 cups (240 g) torn spinach
> 1½ cups each: watermelon (154 g), honeydew (177 g), and cantaloupe balls (177 g)
> ⅓ cup each: thinly sliced cucumber (43 g), red onion (50 g)
> Honey Dressing (recipe follows)

1. Combine all ingredients in salad bowl and toss.

HONEY DRESSING

ABOUT ½ CUP (118 ML)

> 2–3 tablespoons each: (30–45 mL) honey, orange juice, lime juice
> 1–2 tablespoons each (15–30 mL): red wine vinegar, olive oil
> 1 teaspoon (5 mL) dried tarragon leaves
> ⅛ teaspoon (.625 mL) salt

1. Mix all ingredients.

Per Serving: Calories: 85; % of calories from fat: 36; Fat (g): 3.6; Saturated fat (g): 0.5; Cholesterol (mg): 0; Sodium (mg): 50; Protein (g): 1.7; Carbohydrate (g): 13.2; Exchanges: Milk: 0.0; Vegetable: 0.0; Fruit: 1.0; Bread: 0.0; Meat: 0.0; Fat: 0.5

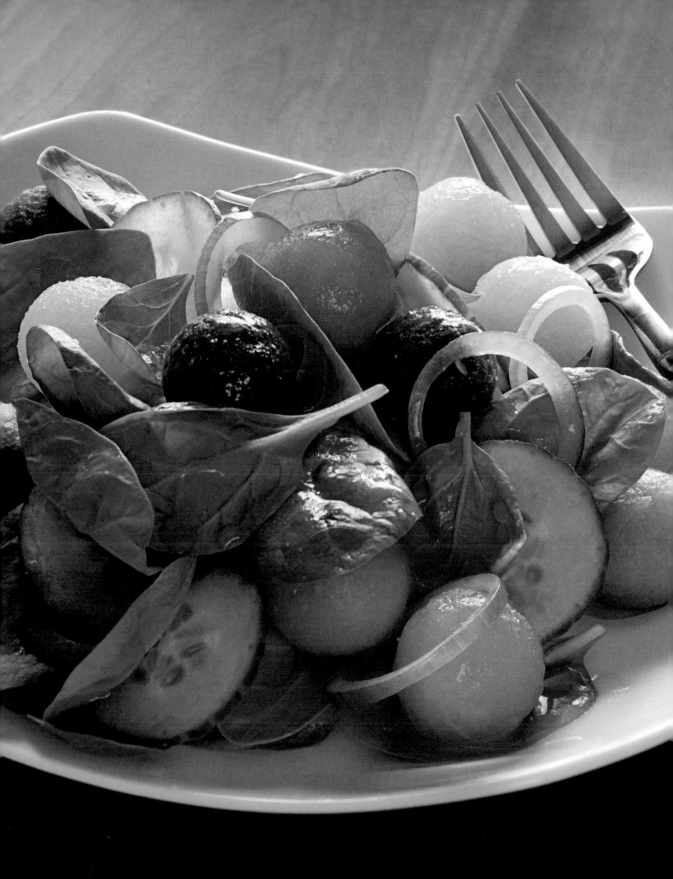

WILTED SPINACH SALAD

A healthful variation of this favorite salad that includes crumbled bacon for traditional flavor.

1 package (10 ounces [280 g]) fresh spinach
4 green onions, sliced
4 slices bacon, cooked crisp, drained, crumbled
1 hard-cooked egg, chopped
1 cup (236 mL) fat-free French or sweet-sour salad dressing
Salt and pepper, to taste

1. Combine the spinach, onions, bacon, and egg in salad bowl.

2. Heat French dressing to boiling in a small saucepan; pour over salad and toss. Season to taste with salt and pepper.

Per Serving: Calories: 95; % of calories from fat: 26; Fat (g): 2.6; Saturated fat (g): 0.8; Cholesterol (mg): 38.2; Sodium (mg): 418; Protein (g): 3.4; Carbohydrate (g): 12.6 Exchanges: Milk: 0.0; Vegetable: 1.0; Fruit: 0.0; Bread: 0.5; Meat: 0.0; Fat: 0.5

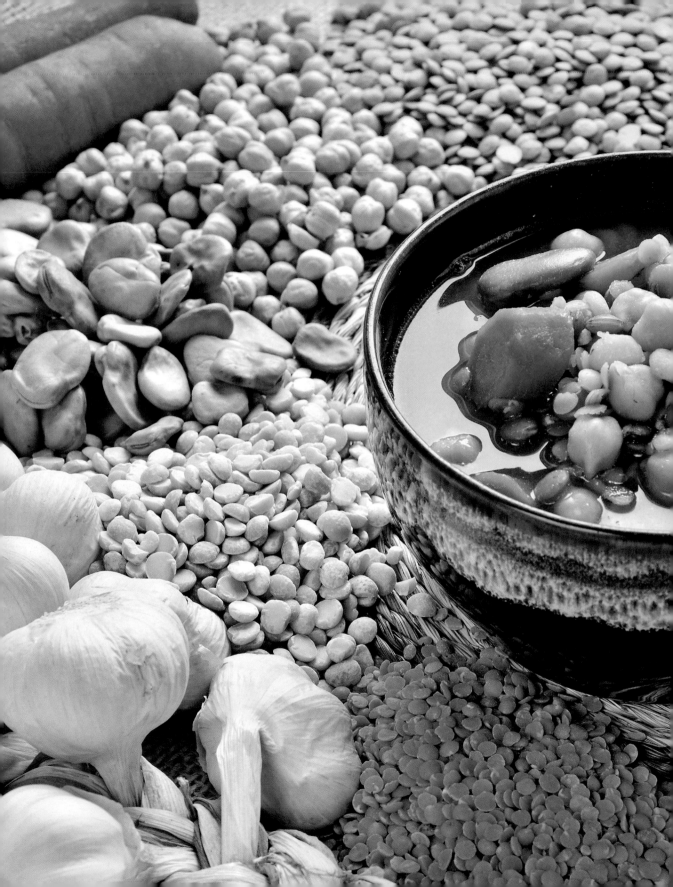

SOUPS

DILLED BEET SOUP

It's not necessary to peel beets, as the skins slip off easily after cooking.

8 FIRST-COURSE SERVINGS (ABOUT 1¼ CUPS [295 ML] EACH)

> **12 medium beets, tops trimmed, scrubbed (about 3 pounds [1.37 kg])**
> **3 cups (708 mL) water**
> **2–3 chicken bouillon cubes**
> **¾–1 cup (178–236 mL) dry red wine or chicken broth**
> **1½–2 teaspoons (7.5–10 mL) dried dill weed**
> **2–3 tablespoons (30–45 mL) red wine vinegar**
> **Salt and pepper, to taste**
> **Thin lemon slices, for garnish**

1. Heat the beets, 3 cups water, and bouillon cubes to boiling in a large saucepan; reduce heat and simmer, covered, until beets are tender, 30 to 40 minutes. Drain, reserving cooking liquid.

2. Slip skins off beets and cut beets into quarters.

3. Add enough water to reserved cooking liquid to make 6 cups (1.4 L). Process the beets, wine, reserved cooking liquid, and dill weed in a food processor or blender until smooth. Season to taste with the vinegar, salt, and pepper. Serve warm or chilled; garnish each bowl of soup with a lemon slice.

Per Serving: **Calories: 63; % of calories from fat: 3; Fat (g): 0.3; Saturated fat (g): 0; Cholesterol (mg): 0; Sodium (mg): 318; Protein (g): 1.8; Carbohydrate (g): 10.6** Exchanges: **Milk: 0.0; Vegetable: 2.0; Fruit: 0.0; Bread: 0.0; Meat: 0.0; Fat: 0.0**

BLACK BEAN SOUP

Minced or whole garlic is available in the vegetable section of large super-markets. Using fresh garlic in this recipe really enhances its flavor. This recipe comes from Diabetes Snacks, Treats, and Easy Eats *by Barbara Grunes.*

10 FIRST-COURSE (1-CUP [236-ML]) SERVINGS

> Olive oil cooking spray
> 1 cup each: chopped onion (150 g), chopped carrot (128 g)
> 1 can (28 ounces [840 mL]) low-sodium chicken broth
> 1 can (14½ ounces [411 g]) low-sodium diced tomatoes, und-rained
> 2 cans (15 ounces [425 g] each) black beans, rinsed, drained, and mashed
> 1 teaspoon (5 mL) minced garlic
> ¼ teaspoon (1.25 ml) each: ground cumin, salt
> ⅛ teaspoon (.625 mL) pepper

1. Lightly coat a large soup pot with cooking spray. Cook the onion and carrot over medium heat for 5 minutes, stirring occasionally. Stir in broth, tomatoes, beans, garlic, cumin, salt, and pepper. Heat to boiling. Reduce heat to a simmer and cook, partially covered, about 10 minutes. Cool slightly.

2. Process the soup in batches in a food processor or blender until smooth. Return soup to pot and heat.

Serving Suggestion: Add dried oregano, dried thyme, and chopped fresh cilantro during cooking for extra flavor. Garnish the soup at the table with chopped white, red, or green onion passed in a small bowl.

Per Serving: **Calories:** 103; **% calories from fat:** 5; **Fat (g):** 0.6; **Saturated fat (g):** 0; **Cholesterol (mg):** 8.3; **Sodium (mg):** 424; **Protein (g):** 7; **Carbohydrate (g):** 16.2
Exchanges: **Milk:** 0.0; **Vegetable:** 0.0; **Fruit:** 0.0; **Bread:** 1.0; **Meat:** 0.5; **Fat:** 0.0

HERBED CUCUMBER SOUP

This soup is very delicate in flavor. Use a serrated grapefruit spoon to seed cucumbers quickly and easily.

6 FIRST-COURSE SERVINGS (ABOUT 1⅓ CUPS [315 ML] EACH)

½ cup (75 g) chopped onion

6 medium cucumbers (about 3 pounds [1.37 kg]), peeled, seeded, chopped

3 tablespoons (23 g) all-purpose flour

4 cups (.95 L) reduced-sodium fat-free chicken broth

1 teaspoon (5 mL) dried mint or dill weed

½ cup (118 mL) fat-free half-and-half or fat-free milk

Salt and white pepper, to taste

Paprika and thin slices cucumber, for garnish

1. Sauté the onion in a lightly greased skillet until tender, 3 to 5 minutes.

2. Add the cucumbers and cook over medium heat 5 minutes; stir in the flour and cook about 1 minute longer. Add the broth and mint to saucepan; heat to boiling. Reduce heat and simmer, covered, 10 minutes.

3. Process the soup in a food processor or blender until smooth; stir in half-and-half and season to taste with salt and pepper. Serve warm or chilled; garnish each bowl of soup with paprika and cucumber slices.

Per Serving: **Calories: 70; % of calories from fat: 8; Fat (g): 0.6; Saturated fat (g): 0.1; Cholesterol (mg): 0; Sodium (mg): 33; Protein (g): 3.1; Carbohydrate (g): 13.7** Exchanges: **Milk: 0.0; Vegetable: 1.0; Fruit: 0.0; Bread: 0.5; Meat: 0.0; Fat: 0.0**

TORTILLA SOUP

For extra zip, add 1 can (4 ounces [114 g]) of drained chopped mild green chilies. Sprinkle the finished soup with a little reduced-fat shredded Monterey Jack cheese or crumbled goat cheese.

6 FIRST-COURSE (2-CUP [473-ML]) SERVINGS

> 1 can (14 ½ ounces [411 g]) low-sodium diced tomatoes, undrained
> 1 cup (100 g) chopped green onions
> 1 tablespoon (15 mL) chopped cilantro
> ½ teaspoon (2.5 mL) garlic powder
> ⅛ teaspoon (.625 mL) each: salt, pepper
> 1 can (48 ounces [1.4 L]) low-sodium chicken broth
> Olive oil cooking spray
> 3 whole wheat 99% fat-free tortillas, cut into strips

1. Using a food processor or blender, pulse the tomatoes and their liquid with the onions, cilantro, garlic powder, salt, and pepper until evenly blended. Pour mixture into a saucepan. Stir in broth.

2. Heat the soup to boiling over medium heat. Partially cover and simmer 5 minutes.

3. While soup cooks, lightly coat a nonstick skillet with cooking spray. Cook the tortilla strips over medium-high heat, stirring often and spraying once, about 2 minutes or just until crisp.

4. Ladle the soup into individual bowls and top with tortilla strips.

Per Serving: **Calories:** 88; **% calories from fat:** 15; **Fat (g):** 1.4; **Saturated fat (g):** 0; **Cholesterol (mg):** 23.6; **Sodium (mg):** 402; **Protein (g):** 8.3; **Carbohydrate (g):** 9.6
Exchanges: **Milk:** 0.0; **Vegetable:** 0.0; **Fruit:** 0.0; **Bread:** 0.5; **Meat:** 0.0; **Fat:** 0.5

TORTELLINI AND MUSHROOM SOUP >

Porcini mushrooms, a Tuscan delicacy abundant in the fall, are available in dried form year round. Porcinis impart a wonderful earthy flavor to recipes. Other dried mushrooms can be substituted for a similar flavor. This recipe comes from 1,001 Delicious Recipes for People with Diabetes *by Sue Spitler.*

6 FIRST-COURSE SERVINGS (ABOUT 1 CUP [236 ML] EACH)

> 1 ounce (28 g) dried porcini mushrooms
> 8 ounces (224 g) fresh white mushrooms, sliced
> 2 tablespoons (30 mL) finely chopped shallots or green onions
> 2 cloves garlic, minced
> ½ teaspoon (2.5 mL) dried tarragon or thyme leaves
> 2 cans (14½ ounces [1.4 L] each) reduced-sodium beef broth
> ¼ cup (59 mL) dry sherry (optional)
> 1 package (9 ounces [255 g]) fresh tomato-and-cheese tortellini
> Salt and pepper, to taste

1. Place the dried mushrooms in bowl; pour hot water over to cover. Let stand until mushrooms are soft, about 15 minutes; drain. Slice mushrooms, discarding any tough parts.

2. Sauté porcini and white mushrooms, shallots, garlic, and tarragon in a lightly greased saucepan until mushrooms are tender, about 5 minutes.

3. Add the broth and sherry and heat to boiling; add the tortellini. Reduce heat and simmer, uncovered, until tortellini are al dente, about 5 minutes; season to taste with salt and pepper.

Per Serving: **Calories: 110**; **% of calories from fat: 16**; **Fat (g): 2**; **Saturated fat (g): 0.4**; **Cholesterol (mg): 4.2**; **Sodium (mg): 184**; **Protein (g): 5**; **Carbohydrate (g): 17.1** Exchanges: **Milk: 0.0**; **Vegetable: 1.0**; **Fruit: 0.0**; **Bread: 1.0**; **Meat: 0.0**; **Fat: 0.5**

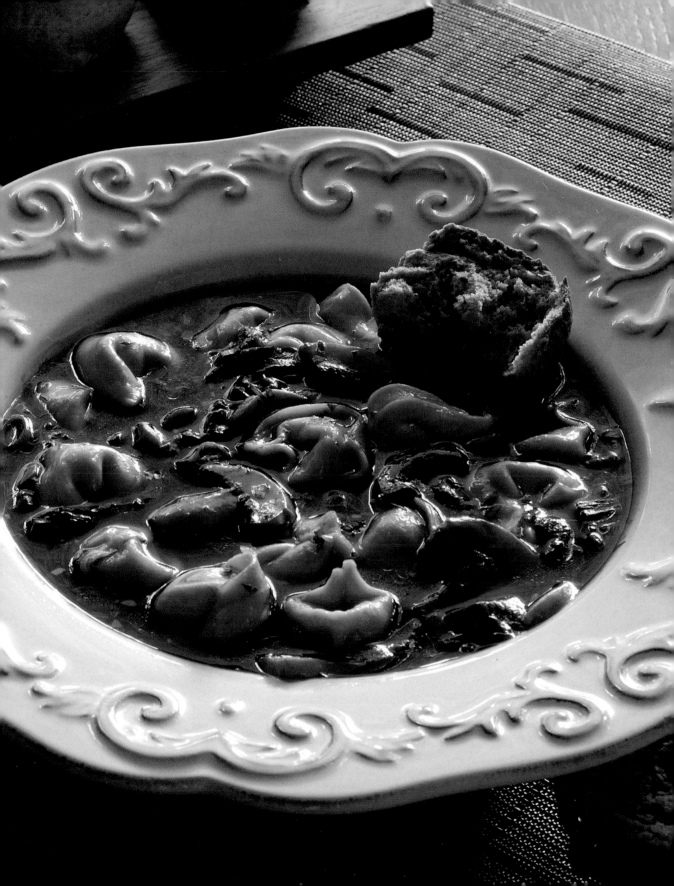

WONTON SOUP

For a complete meal in a bowl, add bits of leftover meat, chicken, and vegetables to Wonton Soup. Add fresh vegetables, such as watercress, snow peas, bamboo shoots, and sliced Chinese cabbage for more flavor.

8 FIRST-COURSE (1-CUP [236-ML]) SERVINGS

> 1 can (48 ounces [1.4 L]) low-sodium chicken broth
> ¼ cup (25 g) chopped green onions
> Vegetable-Filled Wontons (recipe follows)

1. Heat the broth, onions, and wontons to boiling in a large soup pot. Reduce heat to a simmer and cook about 5 minutes, or until hot.

VEGETABLE-FILLED WONTONS

24 WONTONS (8 SERVINGS OF 3)

> Butter-flavored cooking spray
> ½ cup (50 g) chopped green onions
> 2 cups (150 g) chopped white mushrooms
> Salt and pepper, to taste
> 24 wonton wrappers
> 1 egg white, lightly beaten

1. Coat a nonstick skillet with cooking spray. Add the green onions and mushrooms and cook over medium-high heat, stirring occasionally until tender, about 5 minutes. Season to taste with salt and pepper. Cool and drain.

2. To assemble wontons, place 1 scant tablespoon of filling in the center of each wonton wrapper. Brush edges of the wrapper with egg white. Fold the wrapper in half, making a triangular shape, and press along edges, sealing wontons. Set wontons on lightly floured cookie sheet. Cover with plastic wrap to prevent drying.

3. Fill a medium saucepan half-full of water. Heat to boiling. Slide a batch of the wontons into the water. Cook wontons in batches 1½ to 2 minutes, or until wontons are tender. Remove the wontons with a slotted spoon and place in a single layer on a sprayed heated platter.

Per Serving: **Calories: 55;** % calories from fat: 21; **Fat (g): 1.3;** Saturated fat (g): 0; **Cholesterol (mg): 18.7;** Sodium (mg): 210; **Protein (g): 5.9;** Carbohydrate (g): 4.7 Exchanges: **Milk: 0.0;** Vegetable: 1.0; **Fruit: 0.0;** Bread: 0.0; **Meat: 0.0;** Fat: 0.5

PUMPKIN SOUP

This soup has some texture. If you prefer a smooth soup, cool the soup slightly and purée in a blender or food processor. Reheat the soup to serve.

8 FIRST-COURSE (1-CUP [236-ML]) SERVINGS

> Butter-flavored cooking spray
> 1½ cups (225 g) chopped red bell pepper
> 1 medium onion, chopped
> 1 can (29 ounces [822 mL]) pumpkin purée
> 1 can (28 ounces [794 mL]) low-sodium chicken broth
> 1 teaspoon (5 mL) pumpkin pie spice

1. Lightly coat a medium saucepan with cooking spray. Cook the bell pepper and onion over medium heat for 5 minutes, stirring occasionally.

2. Stir in the pumpkin, broth, and spice mixture. Continue cooking for 20 minutes, partially covered.

Per Serving: **Calories: 67;** % calories from fat: 12; **Fat (g): 1;** Saturated fat (g): 0.2; **Cholesterol (mg): 10.3;** Sodium (mg): 110; **Protein (g): 4.4;** Carbohydrate (g): 11.4 Exchanges: **Milk: 0.0;** Vegetable: 0.0; **Fruit: 0.0;** Bread: 1.0; **Meat: 0.0;** Fat: 0.0

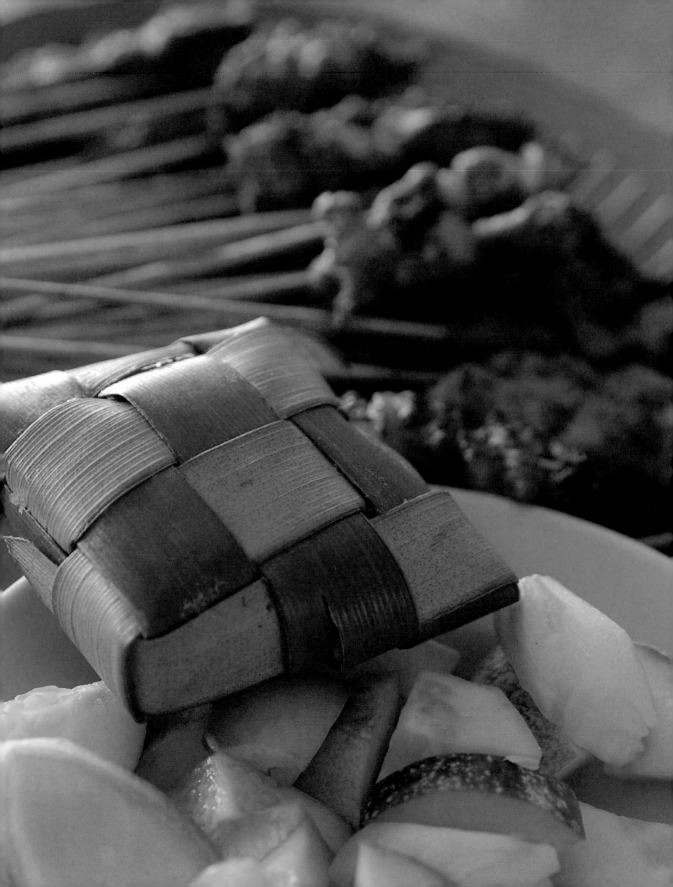

BEEF STEWS AND ENTRÉES

BEEF SATAY

Serve Beef Satay with sliced cucumbers sprinkled with chopped green onions. For extra zip, sprinkle a little mild curry powder on the beef before grilling.

8 SKEWERS (1 SKEWER PER SERVING)

> 1 pound (454 g) beef flank steak or sirloin, cut against the grain into thin slices
> ½ cup (118 mL) fat-free red wine salad dressing
> 6 bamboo skewers, soaked in water 20 minutes

1. Thread the beef slices onto skewers. Place beef skewers into a glass dish and brush with dressing. Marinate, refrigerated, 2 hours. Remove from marinade and drain. Discard marinade.

2. Preheat stovetop or electric indoor grill or broiler. Grill meat a few minutes on each side to desired doneness.

Serving Suggestion: Serve, if desired, with Thai Peanut Sauce (see page 101).

Per Serving: **Calories: 89**; **% calories from fat: 41**; **Fat (g): 3.9**; **Saturated fat (g): 1.7**; **Cholesterol (mg): 22.8**; **Sodium (mg): 50**; **Protein (g): 12.4**; **Carbohydrate (g): 0.1** Exchanges: **Milk: 0.0**; **Vegetable: 0.0**; **Fruit: 0.0**; **Bread: 0.0**; **Meat: 1.5**; **Fat: 0.0**

BEEF AND ANCHO CHILI STEW

This stew has lots of delicious sauce, so serve with crusty warm rolls or tortillas.

8 SERVINGS

> 3 cups (708 mL) boiling water
> 4–6 ancho chilies, stems, seeds, and veins discarded
> 4 medium tomatoes, cut into wedges
> 2 pounds (908 g) beef eye of round, fat trimmed, cubed (¾-inch [2-cm])
> 1 large onion, chopped
> 2 cloves garlic, minced
> 1 teaspoon (5 mL) each: minced jalapeño pepper, dried oregano leaves, crushed cumin seeds
> 2 tablespoons (30 mL) all-purpose flour
> Salt and pepper, to taste

1. Pour boiling water over chilies in bowl; let stand until softened, about 10 minutes. Process chilies and water and tomatoes in blender or food processor until smooth.

2. Sauté beef in a lightly greased Dutch oven until browned, about 5 minutes. Add the onion, garlic, jalapeno pepper, oregano, and cumin; cook until onion is tender, about 5 minutes. Stir in the flour; cook over medium heat 1 minute. Add the ancho chili mixture; heat to boiling. Reduce heat and simmer, covered, until beef is tender, 45 to 60 minutes. Season to taste with salt and pepper.

Per Serving: **Calories: 159; % of calories from fat: 23; Fat (g): 4; Saturated fat (g): 1.3; Cholesterol (mg): 54.7; Sodium (mg): 56; Protein (g): 22.1; Carbohydrate (g): 8.3** Exchanges: **Milk: 0.0; Vegetable: 1.0; Fruit: 0.0; Bread: 0.0; Meat: 2.5; Fat: 0.0**

SHISH KEBABS >

To prevent charring, soak bamboo or wooden skewers in water for 20 minutes before threading on the meat and vegetables. This recipe comes from Diabetes Snacks, Treats, and Easy Eats *by Barbara Grunes.*

4 SKEWERS (1 KEBAB PER SERVING)

> 4 ounces (112 g) beef sirloin steak, trimmed of fat and cut into 1-ounce [28-g] cubes
> 1 cup (236 mL) fat-free Russian salad dressing
> 16 cherry tomatoes
> 2 cups (300 g) square-cut red bell pepper
> 16 mushrooms, stems removed
> 4 wooden, or metal, skewers

1. Toss the steak with dressing in a glass bowl. Cover with plastic wrap and refrigerate overnight, turning steak once or twice.

2. Just before cooking, remove the steak from the marinade. Discard marinade.

3. Thread skewers with meat, tomatoes, bell peppers, and mushrooms.

4. Preheat an outdoor grill, stovetop or electric indoor grill, or broiler. Cook kebabs, turning every 4 minutes, until beef is cooked to desired doneness.

Serving Suggestion: Serve kebabs wrapped in whole wheat pita pockets or with whole-grain couscous, if your eating plan allows.

Per Serving: **Calories: 99**; **% calories from fat: 16**; **Fat (g): 1.9**; **Saturated fat (g): 0.5**; **Cholesterol (mg): 17.2**; **Sodium (mg): 84**; **Protein (g): 9.4**; **Carbohydrate (g): 13.1** Exchanges: **Milk: 0.0**; **Vegetable: 2.0**; **Fruit: 0.0**; **Bread: 0.0**; **Meat: 1.0**; **Fat: 0.0**

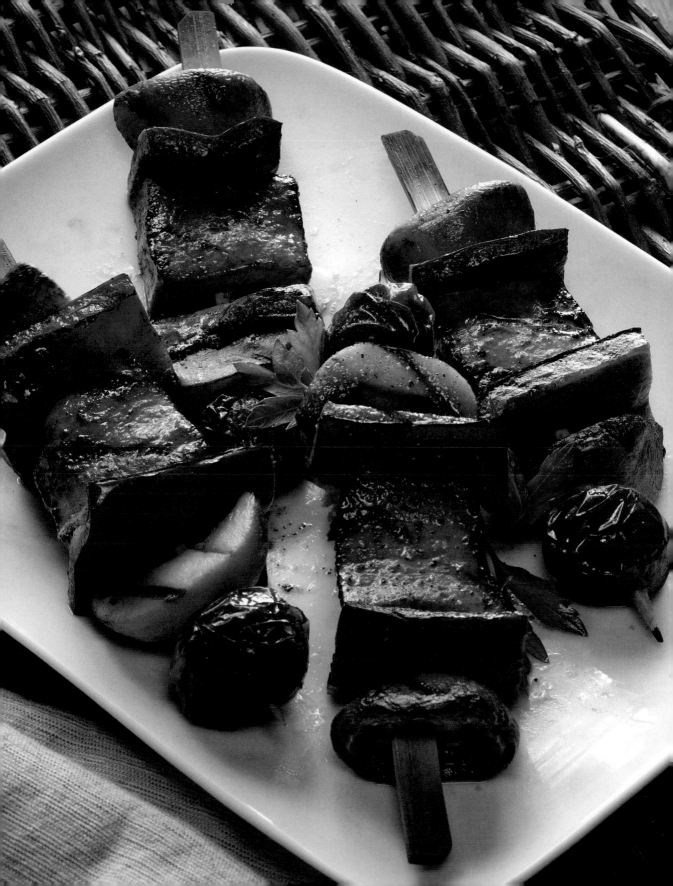

JUST PLAIN MEAT LOAF

Moist, the way meatloaf should be, with plenty of leftovers for sandwiches, too! This recipe comes from 1,001 Delicious Recipes for People with Diabetes *by Sue Spitler.*

6 SERVINGS

> 1½ pounds (680 g) very lean ground beef
> 1 cup (90 g) quick-cooking oats
> ½ cup (118 mL) fat-free milk
> 1 egg
> ¼ cup (59 mL) ketchup or chili sauce
> ½ cup each: chopped onion (75 g), green bell pepper (75 g)
> 1 teaspoon (5 mL) each: minced garlic, dried Italian seasoning
> ¾ teaspoon (3.75 mL) salt
> ½ teaspoon (2.5 mL) pepper

1. Mix all ingredients until blended. Pat mixture into an ungreased loaf pan, 9 × 5 inches (22.5 cm × 13 cm), or shape into a loaf in baking pan.

2. Bake at 350°F (180°C) until juices run clear and meat thermometer registers 170°F (77°C), about 1 hour. Let stand in pan 10 minutes; invert onto a serving plate.

VARIATIONS

Stuffed Green Peppers—Cut 6 medium green bell peppers lengthwise into halves; discard seeds. Cook peppers in simmering water 3 minutes; drain. Make recipe as above, substituting 1 cup (160 g) cooked rice for the oats. Fill peppers with mixture and place in baking pan. Bake, covered, at 350°F (180°C) until beef mixture is cooked, about 45 minutes.

Italian Meat Loaf—Make recipe as above, adding ¼ cup (1 ounce [28 g]) grated fat-free Parmesan cheese, ½ cup (2 ounces [56 g]) shredded reduced-fat mozzarella cheese, and 2 tablespoons (30 mL) chopped pitted black olives. After baking, spread meat loaf with 2 tablespoons (30 mL) seasoned tomato sauce and sprinkle with 2 tablespoons (30 mL) each fat-free Parmesan and shredded reduced-fat mozzarella cheeses. Let stand, loosely covered, 10 minutes.

Savory Cheese Meat Loaf—Make recipe as above, substituting ½ pound (224 g) ground lean pork for ½ pound (224 g) of the beef, and adding 4 ounces (112 g) fat-free cream cheese, ½ cup (2 ounces [56 g]) shredded reduced-fat Cheddar cheese, and 2 table-spoons (30 mL) Worcestershire sauce. Spread top of loaf with ¼ cup (59 mL) of ketchup before baking. Sprinkle ¼ cup (1 ounce [56 g]) shredded reduced-fat Cheddar cheese on top of meat loaf after baking. Let stand, loosely covered, 10 minutes.

Chutney-Peanut Meat Loaf—Make recipe as above, substituting ½ cup (118 mL) chopped chutney for the ketchup, and adding ⅓ cup (53 g) chopped peanuts, 1 teaspoon (5 mL) curry powder, and ½ teaspoon (2.5 mL) ground ginger.

Per Serving: **Calories: 241**; **% of calories from fat: 21**; **Fat (g): 5.5**; **Saturated fat (g): 1.8**; **Cholesterol (mg): 64.3**; **Sodium (mg): 489**; **Protein (g): 31.2**; **Carbohydrate (g): 15.3** Exchanges: **Milk: 0.0**; **Vegetable: 0.0**; **Fruit: 0.0**; **Bread: 1.0**; **Meat: 3.0**; **Fat: 0.0**

BEEF STEAKS WITH TOMATILLO AND AVOCADO SAUCE

The Tomatillo and Avocado Sauce is also excellent with grilled or roasted poultry or pork.

6 SERVINGS

> 1 medium onion, thinly sliced
> 6 beef eye of round or tenderloin steaks (4 ounces [112 g] each), fat trimmed
> Salt and pepper, to taste
> 1 cup (236 mL) Tomatillo Sauce (½ recipe)
> ¼ cup (59 mL) each: mashed avocado, fat-free sour cream
> 6 flour or corn tortillas, warm

1. Sauté the onion in a lightly greased large skillet 2 to 3 minutes; reduce heat to medium-low and cook until onion is very soft, 5 to 8 minutes. Remove from skillet.

2. Add steaks to skillet; cook over medium heat to desired degree of doneness, 3 to 4 minutes on each side for medium. Season to taste with salt and pepper.

3. Heat Tomatillo Sauce in a small saucepan until hot. Stir in the avocado and sour cream; cook 2 minutes. Top steaks with onions and sauce. Serve with tortillas.

TOMATILLO SAUCE

ABOUT 2 CUPS (473 ML)

> 1½ pounds (680 g) Mexican green tomatoes (tomatillos)
> ½ medium onion, chopped
> 1 clove garlic, minced
> ½ small serrano chili, minced
> 3 tablespoons (3 g) finely chopped cilantro
> Vegetable cooking spray
> 2–3 teaspoons sugar
> Salt and white pepper, to taste

1. Remove and discard husks from tomatoes; simmer tomatoes, covered, in 1 inch water in large saucepan until tender, 5 to 8 minutes. Cool; drain.

2. Process tomatoes, onion, garlic, serrano chili, and cilantro in food processor or blender, using pulse technique, until almost smooth. Spray large skillet with cooking spray; heat over medium heat until hot. Add sauce and "fry" over medium heat until slightly thickened, about 5 minutes; season to taste with sugar, salt, and pepper.

Per Serving: **Calories: 271; % of calories from fat: 30; Fat (g): 8.9; Saturated fat (g): 3.1; Cholesterol (mg): 56.3; Sodium (mg): 101; Protein (g): 28.2; Carbohydrate (g): 19.2** Exchanges: **Milk: 0.0; Vegetable: 1.0; Fruit: 0.0; Bread: 1.0; Meat: 3.0; Fat: 0.0**

STEAK AU POIVRE >

Beef eye of round steak is a healthy choice for this entrée, as less than 30% of its calories come from fat.

4 teaspoons (20 mL) coarsely crushed black peppercorns

4 beef eye of round or tenderloin steaks (4 ounces [112 g] each), fat trimmed

Salt

⅓ cup (79 mL) brandy or beef broth

¼ cup (59 mL) apricot preserves

2–4 tablespoons (30–60 mL) spicy brown mustard

2–3 teaspoons (30–45 mL) reduced-sodium Worcester-shire sauce

1 tablespoon (15 mL) each: light brown sugar, prepared horseradish

1 teaspoon (5 mL) each: crushed caraway seeds and black peppercorns

¼ teaspoon (1.25 mL) ground allspice

1. Mix all the ingredients, except beef; spread mixture on beef.

2. Place beef on rack in roasting pan; roast at 325°F (165°C) to desired doneness, 160°F (70°C) for medium, 45 to 60 minutes. Let stand 10 minutes before slicing.

VARIATION

Crumb-Crusted Roast Beef—In place of round or tenderloin steaks, use 1 boneless beef sirloin tip roast, fat trimmed (about 2 pounds [908 g]). Make recipe as above omitting brown sugar, horseradish, caraway seeds, peppercorns, and allspice. Combine 1 cup (60 g) fresh bread crumbs, 2 teaspoons (10 mL) minced garlic,

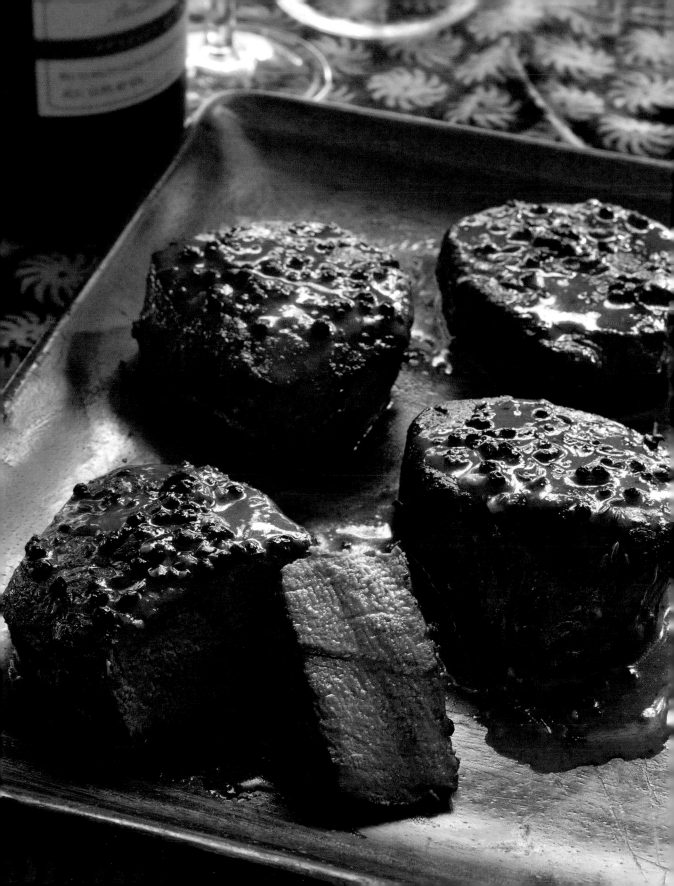

1 teaspoon (5 mL) dried basil leaves, ½ teaspoon (2.5 mL) dried oregano leaves, and ¼ teaspoon (1.25 mL) dried marjoram leaves with the apricot preserves, mustard, and Worcestershire sauce; pat onto beef. Roast as above.

Per Serving: **Calories: 264**; % of calories from fat: 26; **Fat (g): 7.3**; **Saturated fat (g): 2.5**; **Cholesterol (mg): 71.8**; **Sodium (mg): 185**; **Protein (g): 33.9**; **Carbohydrate (g): 12.5**; Exchanges: **Milk: 0.0**; **Vegetable: 0.0**; **Fruit: 0.5**; **Bread: 0.0**; **Meat: 4.0**; **Fat: 0.0**

FLANK STEAK ON SALAD GREENS

For easier slicing, use a Japanese trick and chill the meat in the freezer, nearly to the point of freezing, and always cut against the grain.

8 SERVINGS

> 8 cups (240 g) assorted greens or spinach, washed and drained
> Olive oil cooking spray
> 1 bunch asparagus, bottom ends trimmed
> 2 cups (320 g) sliced tomatoes
> ¾ cup (177 mL) low-calorie balsamic vinaigrette dressing, divided
> 1 pound (454 g) lean flank steak, sliced

1. Arrange the greens on 8 dinner plates.

2. Lightly coat a nonstick indoor electric or stovetop grill or nonstick skillet with cooking spray and preheat. Grill or pan fry the asparagus over medium heat, about 4 minutes or until slightly browned and tender-crisp. Cut asparagus in 2-inch (5-cm) pieces and scatter over the greens. Arrange tomatoes over the asparagus. Drizzle ½ cup (118 mL) dressing equally over salads.

3. Brush the steak slices with the remaining ¼ cup vinaigrette. Grill or pan fry the steak 5 to 7 minutes or until desired doneness. Arrange the steak over the salads.

VARIATION

Grilled Lamb on Salad Greens—For a Russian or Middle Eastern flavor, substitute lean leg of lamb for the beef.

Per Serving: **Calories: 119; % calories from fat: 31; Fat (g): 4.1; Saturated fat (g): 1.7; Cholesterol (mg): 22.8; Sodium (mg): 330; Protein (g): 14.6; Carbohydrate (g): 6.3** Exchanges: **Milk: 0.0; Vegetable: 1.0; Fruit: 0.0; Bread: 0.0; Meat: 2.0; Fat: 0.0**

SOFT TACOS

White or yellow corn tortillas can be substituted for flour tortillas.

6 SERVINGS

> 6 flour tortillas (6 inches [15 cm] in diameter)
> Olive oil cooking spray
> ¼ cup (38 g) chopped onion
> 1 teaspoon (5 mL) chili powder or more to taste
> 6 ounces (170 g) lean ground beef (85% lean)
> 1½ cups (54 g) chopped romaine lettuce
> ¾ cup (120 g) chopped tomato
> 4 ounces (112 g) reduced-fat Cheddar cheese
> ¾ cup (177 mL) fat-free plain yogurt

1. Sprinkle each tortilla lightly with water. Wrap tortillas in foil and place in a 325°F (165°C) oven.

2. Heat a nonstick skillet coated with olive oil cooking spray over medium heat. Add the onion and season with chili powder. Mix in the meat and cook until no longer pink. Drain off any fat.

3. Remove tortillas from the oven. Divide the beef mixture equally among the tortillas. Top with lettuce, tomato, cheese, and yogurt. Fold tortillas in half.

Per Serving: **Calories: 254; % calories from fat: 39; Fat (g): 10.9; Saturated fat (g): 5; Cholesterol (mg): 33; Sodium (mg): 363; Protein (g): 15.1; Carbohydrate (g): 22.7** Exchanges: **Milk: 0.0; Vegetable: 0.0; Fruit: 0.0; Bread: 1.5; Meat: 1.5; Fat: 1.5**

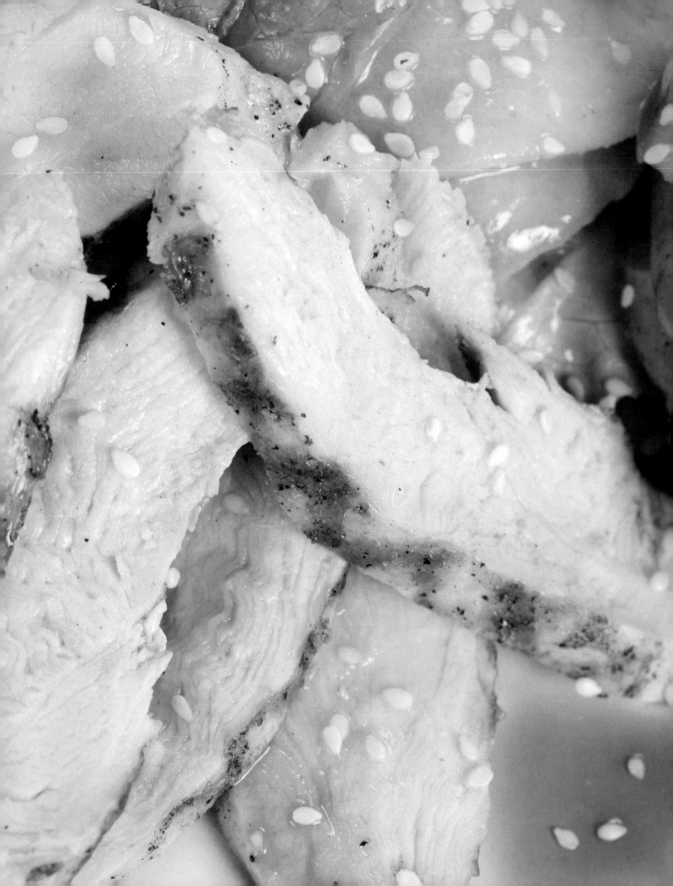

POULTRY STEWS AND ENTRÉES

CHICKEN WITH GINGERED HONEY-ORANGE SAUCE

The sauce combines gingerroot, honey, and orange for delicious flavor. This recipe comes from 1,001 Delicious Recipes for People with Diabetes *by Sue Spitler.*

8 SERVINGS

> 8 skinless chicken breast halves (6 ounces [170 g] each)
> Vegetable oil cooking spray
> Paprika, salt, and pepper
> Gingered Honey-Orange Sauce (recipe follows)

1. Place the chicken in a greased baking pan; spray lightly with cooking spray and sprinkle with paprika, salt and pepper.

2. Bake, uncovered, at 350°F (180°C) until chicken is browned and juices run clear, 30 to 40 minutes, basting occasionally with Gingered Honey-Orange Sauce. Serve with remaining sauce.

GINGERED HONEY-ORANGE SAUCE

ABOUT 1¼ CUPS (295 ML)

> 1 cup (236 mL) orange juice
> 2 tablespoons (30 mL) honey
> Grated zest of 1 orange
> 1–2 tablespoons (15–30 mL) finely chopped gingerroot
> 1 tablespoon (15 mL) all-purpose flour
> 1 orange, peeled, cut into segments

1. Combine all ingredients, except orange segments, in small saucepan; heat to boiling. Boil, whisking until thickened, about 1 minute; stir in orange segments and cook over low heat 2 to 3 minutes.

Per Serving: **Calories: 220; % of calories from fat: 9; Fat (g): 2.1; Saturated fat (g): 0.5; Cholesterol (mg): 99; Sodium (mg): 89; Protein (g): 39.6; Carbohydrate (g): 8.4** Exchanges: **Milk: 0.0; Vegetable: 0.0; Fruit: 0.5; Bread: 0.0; Meat: 5.0; Fat: 0.0**

BBQ CHICKEN BREASTS

For a delicious dinner, serve BBQ Chicken Breasts with Coleslaw (see recipe on page 41) and Corn Bread (see recipe on page 117).

6 SERVINGS (ABOUT 3 OUNCES [85 G] CHICKEN PER SERVING)

> **Butter-flavored cooking spray**
> **1 pound (454 g) boneless, skinless chicken breast halves (about 4)**
> **½ cup (120 mL) Barbecue Sauce (see recipe on page 100) or store-bought**

1. Lightly coat a shallow baking pan with cooking spray.

2. Place chicken in the pan and brush with half of the sauce. Cover with foil and bake at 425°F (220°C) 35 minutes.

3. Uncover and bake until the chicken is no longer pink in the center, about 10 minutes. Brush with remaining sauce. Remove from oven and slice into 6 portions.

Per Serving: **Calories: 98; % calories from fat: 12; Fat (g): 1.3; Saturated fat (g): 0.3; Cholesterol (mg): 43.8; Sodium (mg): 209; Protein (g): 17.8; Carbohydrate (g): 2.7** Exchanges: **Milk: 0.0; Vegetable: 0.0; Fruit: 0.0; Bread: 0.0; Meat: 2.0; Fat: 0.0**

CALIFORNIA NO-BEAN CHILI >

This chili sports some California-style touches!

6 SERVINGS

- 1 pound (454 g) boneless, skinless chicken breast, in 1-inch (2.5-cm) cubes
- 1 teaspoon (5 mL) crushed mixed peppercorns
- 4 cups (0.95 L) sliced plum tomatoes
- 1 cup each: diced sun-dried tomatoes (not in oil) (112 g), Zinfandel or other dry red wine (236 mL)
- 2 dried California chilies, chopped
- 4 teaspoons (20 mL) chili powder
- 1 avocado, chopped
- 2 tablespoons (30 mL) sunflower seeds, toasted
- Salt, to taste
- 6 tablespoons (12 g) chopped basil

1. Sauté the chicken and peppercorns in a lightly greased large saucepan until browned, 8 to 10 minutes. Add plum and sun-dried tomatoes, wine, chilies, and chili powder; heat to boiling. Reduce heat and simmer, covered, 10 minutes; simmer, uncovered, until thickened to desired consistency, 5 to 10 minutes. Stir in avocado and sunflower seeds; season to taste with salt. Sprinkle each bowl of chili with basil.

Per Serving: **Calories:** 258; **% of calories from fat:** 30; **Fat (g):** 9.2; **Saturated fat (g):** 1.8; **Cholesterol (mg):** 46; **Sodium (mg):** 272; **Protein (g):** 21.5; **Carbohydrate (g):** 19.7 Exchanges: **Milk:** 0.0; **Vegetable:** 4.0; **Fruit:** 0.0; **Bread:** 0.0; **Meat:** 2.0; **Fat:** 1.0

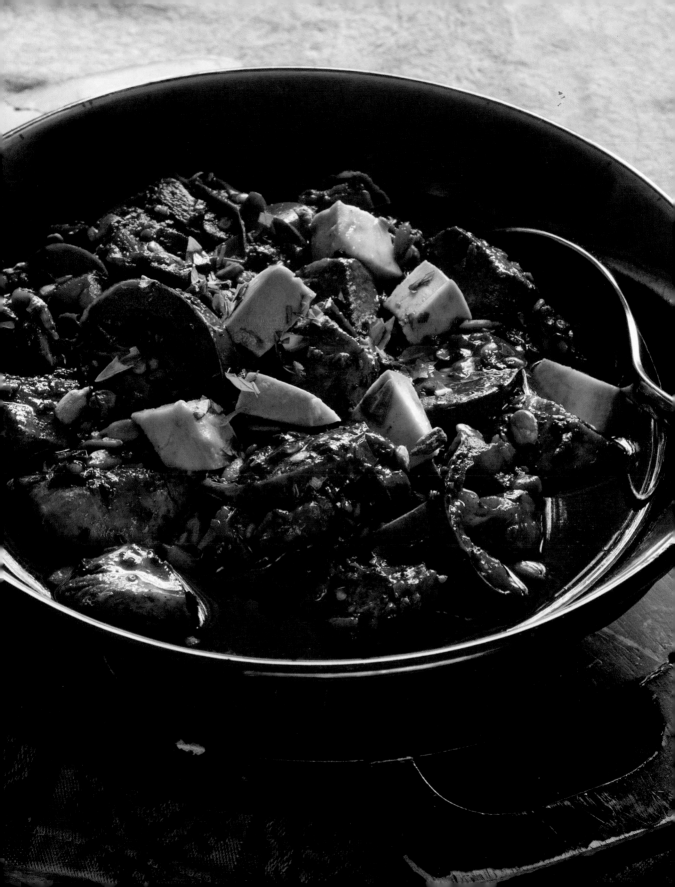

CHICKEN BREASTS WITH ROSEMARY

Easy, yet elegant, this healthful entrée is good served with a simple vegetable or salad.

4 SERVINGS

> 1 tablespoon (15 mL) olive oil
>
> 1½ teaspoons (7.5 mL) balsamic vinegar
>
> 1 teaspoon (5 mL) minced garlic
>
> 1 tablespoon (30 mL) grated lemon zest
>
> ¼ teaspoon (1.25 mL) each: salt, pepper
>
> 4 boneless, skinless chicken breast halves (4 ounces [112 g] each)
>
> ½–¾ cup (118–177 mL) dry white wine or reduced-sodium chicken broth
>
> ½ cup (80 g) chopped tomato
>
> 1 teaspoon (5 mL) finely chopped fresh or ½ teaspoon (2.5 mL) dried rosemary leaves

1. Brush the combined olive oil, vinegar, garlic, lemon zest, salt, and pepper over the chicken; let stand 10 minutes. Cook the chicken in a lightly greased large skillet over medium heat until browned, about 5 minutes on each side. Add the wine, tomato, and rosemary to the skillet and heat to boiling; reduce heat and simmer, covered, until chicken is cooked, about 15 minutes.

Per Serving: **Calories:** 188; **% of calories from fat:** 31; **Fat (g):** 6.4; **Saturated fat (g):** 1.3; **Cholesterol (mg):** 69; **Sodium (mg):** 209; **Protein (g):** 25.6; **Carbohydrate (g):** 2.6 Exchanges: **Milk:** 0.0; **Vegetable:** 0.5; **Fruit:** 0.0; **Bread:** 0.0; **Meat:** 3.0; **Fat:** 0.0

ARROZ CON POLLO

4 SERVINGS

Olive oil cooking spray

4 boneless, skinless chicken breasts

1 cup each: sliced onion (150 g) and green bell pepper (150 g), chopped seeded tomato (160 g), uncooked rice (190 g)

½ cup (118 mL) chicken broth, or as needed

1 (10-ounce [280-g]) package frozen green peas

1. Spray a large nonstick skillet with cooking spray. Add chicken pieces. Cook over medium heat until chicken is done, 10 minutes. Cool slightly and slice thin.

2. Spray and reheat skillet until hot. Stir in onion, bell pepper, tomato, and rice. Cook 5 minutes, stirring often. Add chicken broth and peas. Cover, reduce heat. Simmer 10 minutes, or until rice is tender. Stir in chicken pieces. Serve hot.

Per Serving: **Calories: 322; % calories from fat: 4.2; Fat (g): 1.5; Saturated fat (g): 0.4; Cholesterol (mg): 34.5; Sodium (mg): 216.6; Protein (g): 21.8; Carbohydrate (g): 54.4** Exchanges: **Milk: 0.0; Vegetable: 0.0; Fruit: 0.0; Bread: 3.0; Meat: 2.0; Fat: 0.0**

CHICKEN CORDON BLEU >

A favorite gourmet entrée, the ham and cheese-stuffed chicken breasts are delicious in their new low-fat form!

6 SERVINGS

> 6 boneless, skinless chicken breast halves (4 ounces [112 g] each)
>
> 4 ounces (112 g) sliced fat-free Swiss cheese
>
> 3 ounces (85 g) lean smoked ham
>
> All-purpose flour
>
> 1 egg, lightly beaten
>
> ⅓ cup (50 g) unseasoned dry bread crumbs
>
> Vegetable oil cooking spray

1. Pound the chicken breasts with the flat side of a meat mallet until very thin and even in thickness. Layer the cheese and ham on the chicken, cutting to fit; roll up and secure with toothpicks.

2. Coat chicken rolls lightly with flour; dip in egg and coat with bread crumbs. Spray rolls generously with cooking spray and cook in large ovenproof skillet over medium heat until browned on all sides, 8 to 10 minutes. Transfer to oven and bake at 350°F (180°C), uncovered, until cooked, about 25 minutes.

Per Serving: **Calories:** 210; **% of calories from fat:** 18; **Fat (g):** 3.9; **Saturated fat (g):** 1.1; **Cholesterol (mg):** 73.2; **Sodium (mg):** 540; **Protein (g):** 34.6; **Carbohydrate (g):** 6.3 Exchanges: **Milk:** 0.0; **Vegetable:** 0.0; **Fruit:** 0.0; **Bread:** 0.0; **Meat:** 4.0; **Fat:** 0.0

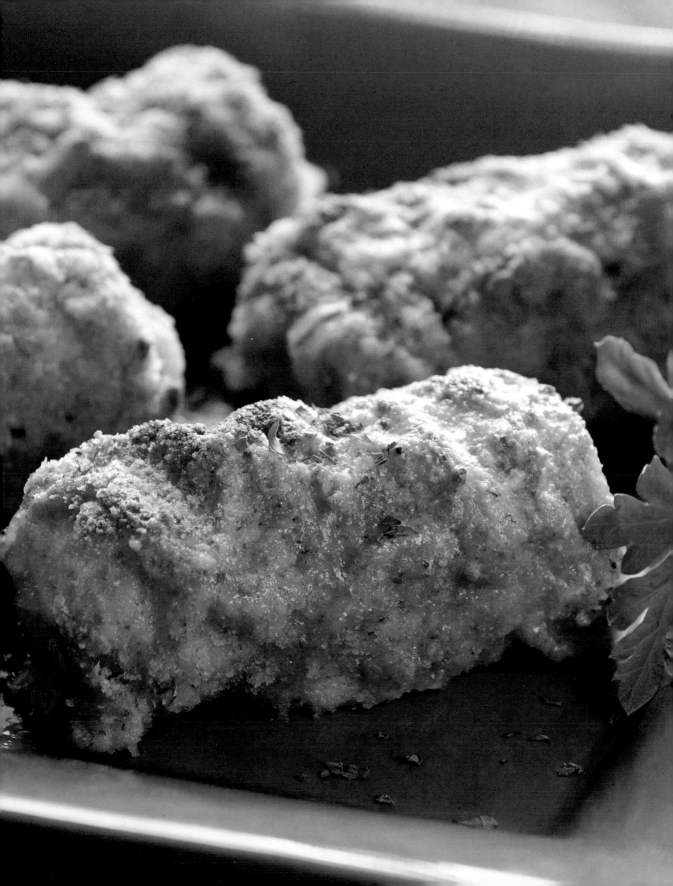

OVEN-FRIED CHICKEN DRUMSTICKS

This is great for a children's party. Use small drumsticks to maintain portion control. This recipe comes from Diabetes Snacks, Treats, and Easy Eats *by Barbara Grunes.*

8 SERVINGS (1 DRUMSTICK PER SERVING)

> **Butter-flavored cooking spray**
> **8 small chicken drumsticks, skin removed**
> **1 cup (60 g) crushed whole-grain cereal**
> **⅓ cup (79 mL) egg substitute**

1. Lightly coat a baking sheet with cooking spray.

2. Rinse chicken and pat dry with paper towels. Put cereal on a piece of wax paper and the egg substitute in a shallow bowl. Roll each drumstick in egg substitute and then in crumbs. Press crumbs into drumsticks.

3. Place drumsticks on baking sheet. Bake at 400°F (200°C) until chicken is no longer pink and juices run clear, 45 minutes. Let chicken cool for 5 minutes before serving.

Per Serving: **Calories: 118**; **% calories from fat: 18**; **Fat (g): 2.3**; **Saturated fat (g): 0.5**; **Cholesterol (mg): 43.6**; **Sodium (mg): 138**; **Protein (g): 13.5**; **Carbohydrate (g): 9.7** Exchanges: **Milk: 0.0**; **Vegetable: 0.0**; **Fruit: 0.0**; **Bread: 0.5**; **Meat: 1.5**; **Fat: 0.0**

CHICKEN AND CHEESE RELLENOS

Our healthy version of chili rellenos eliminates the customary egg coating and frying in oil.

6 SERVINGS

> 6 large poblano chili peppers
> 1 each: chopped medium onion, carrot, garlic clove
> 1 pound (454 g) boneless, skinless chicken breast, cooked, shredded
> ⅓ cup (80 g) whole kernel corn
> ½ teaspoon (2.5 mL) each: ground cumin, dried thyme leaves
> ½ cup (2 ounces [56 g]) each: shredded reduced-fat Monterey Jack, fat-free Cheddar cheese
> Salt and pepper, to taste
> 1 tablespoon (15 mL) vegetable oil
> Chili Tomato Sauce (recipe follows)

1. Cut the stems from tops of chili peppers; remove and discard seeds and veins. Simmer the peppers in water to cover until slightly softened, 2 to 3 minutes; drain and cool.

2. Sauté the onion, carrot, and garlic in a lightly greased large skillet until tender, 3 to 5 minutes. Add the chicken, corn, cumin and thyme; cook over medium heat 1 to 2 minutes. Remove from heat and stir in the cheeses; season to taste with salt and pepper.

3. Spoon the mixture into the peppers; sauté in oil in large skillet until tender and browned on all sides, 6 to 8 minutes. Serve with Chili Tomato Sauce.

CHILI TOMATO SAUCE

1 CUP (236 ML)

> 1 cup (236 mL) reduced-sodium tomato sauce
> 2 tablespoons (30 mL) water
> 1–1½ tablespoons (15–22 mL) chili powder
> 1 clove garlic
> Salt and pepper, to taste

1. Heat all ingredients, except the salt and pepper, to boiling in a small saucepan; reduce heat and simmer, uncovered, 2 to 3 minutes. Season to taste with salt and pepper.

Per Serving: **Calories: 215; % of calories from fat: 26; Fat (g): 6.4; Saturated fat (g): 1.9; Cholesterol (mg): 54.4; Sodium (mg): 213; Protein (g): 25.2; Carbohydrate (g): 15.1** Exchanges: **Milk: 0.0; Vegetable: 2.0; Fruit: 0.0; Bread: 0.5; Meat: 3.0; Fat: 0.0**

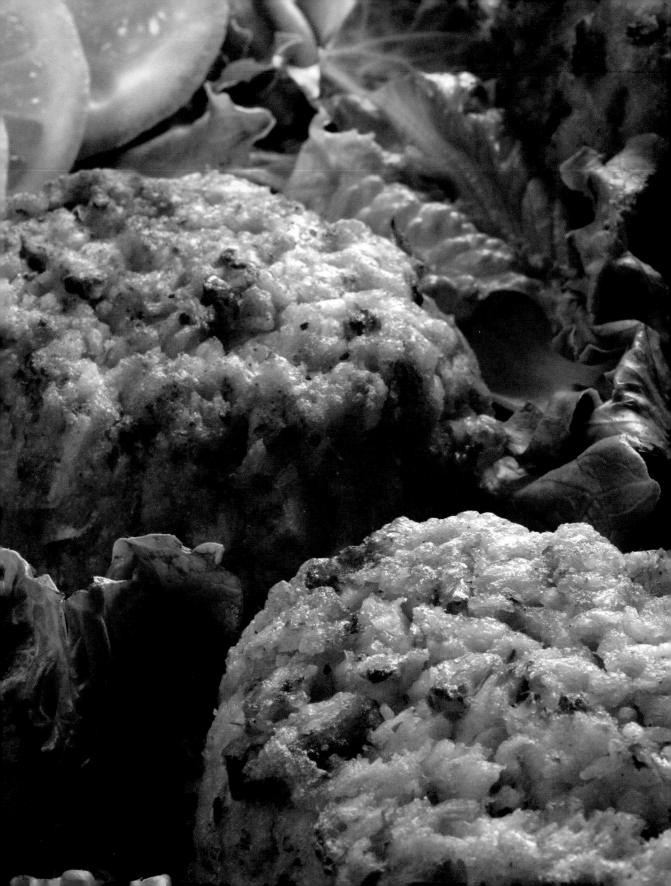

FISH AND SEAFOOD ENTRÉES

CRAB CAKES

Serve these crab cakes with lemon wedges and low-fat tartar sauce.

4 CRAB CAKES (1 PER SERVING)

¼ cup (59 mL) egg substitute
2 tablespoons (30 mL) fat-free mayonnaise
1 teaspoon (5 mL) dry mustard
2 cans (4¼ ounces [120 g] each) crabmeat, or fresh crab-
    meat, about ½ pound (227 g)
¾ cup (45 g) fresh whole wheat bread crumbs
Salt, to taste
⅛ teaspoon (.625 mL) pepper
Butter-flavored cooking spray

1. Beat together the egg substitute, mayonnaise, and mustard
    in a large bowl. Stir in the crabmeat, crumbs, salt, and pep-
    per.

2. Shape the mixture into 4 cakes. Place the cakes on a plate
    and cover lightly with plastic wrap. Refrigerate at least 1
    hour to firm up cakes.

3. Lightly coat a nonstick skillet with cooking spray. Fry the
    cakes over medium heat, turning once, 3 to 4 minutes on
    each side.

Per Serving: **Calories: 69; % calories from fat: 12; Fat (g): 0.9; Saturated fat (g): 0.2;
Cholesterol (mg): 26.8; Sodium (mg): 344; Protein (g): 6.5; Carbohydrate (g): 8.1**
Exchanges: **Milk: 0.0; Vegetable: 0.0; Fruit: 0.0; Bread: 0.5; Meat: 1.0; Fat: 0.0**

SCALLOPS WITH ASPARAGUS

This is an easy dish to make for a last-minute dinner. If you wish, sub-stitute peeled shrimp for the scallops, or use a mixture.

4 (1½-CUP [354-ML]) SERVINGS

> Canola oil cooking spray
> ½ cup (50 g) chopped green onions
> 1 pound (454 g) asparagus, stems trimmed, cut into
>   1½-inch (4-cm) pieces
> ¾ pound (340 g) small scallops
> ¼ cup (59 mL) store-bought stir-fry sauce

1. Lightly coat a large nonstick skillet or wok with cooking spray. Cook the green onions and asparagus, stirring constantly, about 2 minutes.

2. Add the scallops and sauce. Continue cooking and stirring until the scallops are opaque and firm to the touch, about 2 minutes.

Note: Stir-fry sauce is available in the Asian section of most super-markets and in specialty markets.

Per Serving: **Calories: 125; % calories from fat: 6; Fat (g): 0.9; Saturated fat (g): 0.1; Cholesterol (mg): 28.1; Sodium (mg): 661; Protein (g): 17.6; Carbohydrate (g): 12.1** Exchanges: **Milk: 0.0; Vegetable: 2.0; Fruit: 0.0; Bread: 0.0; Meat: 2.0; Fat: 0.0**

SCALLOPS WITH APPLES AND PEA PODS

This colorful dish with an apple accent is delicious served over steamed rice, rice noodles, or Chinese egg noodles. This recipe comes from 1,001 Delicious Recipes for People with Diabetes by Sue Spitler.

4 SERVINGS

3 small apples, unpeeled, thinly sliced
1 each: chopped medium onion, red bell pepper
3 ounces (85 g) snow peas, trimmed
2 tablespoons (30 mL) vegetable oil, divided
12 ounces (341 g) scallops
¼ cup (59 mL) apple cider
2 teaspoons (10 mL) cornstarch
1 tablespoon (15 mL) reduced-sodium soy sauce
Salt and pepper, to taste

1. Stir-fry the apples, onion, bell pepper, and snow peas in 1 tablespoon oil in a wok or large skillet over medium-high heat until crisp-tender, about 3 minutes. Remove from the wok. Add the scallops and stir-fry in remaining 1 tablespoon oil until cooked and opaque, about 4 minutes.

2. Stir in the combined cider, cornstarch, and soy sauce, and cook until the mixture boils and thickens, about 1 minute. Stir in the apple mixture; stir-fry 2 minutes. Season to taste with salt and pepper.

Per Serving: **Calories: 238; % of calories from fat: 30; Fat (g): 8.3; Saturated fat (g): 1; Cholesterol (mg): 36.2; Sodium (mg): 315; Protein (g): 17.5; Carbohydrate (g): 26** Exchanges: **Milk: 0.0; Vegetable: 0.0; Fruit: 1.5; Bread: 0.0; Meat: 2.0; Fat: 1.0**

BRAISED FISH WITH SUN-DRIED TOMATO SAUCE

The combination of tomato sauce and sun-dried tomatoes gives this dish rich tomato flavor. Red snapper or other firm fish can be substituted for the halibut.

4 SERVINGS

> 1 large onion, chopped
> 1 teaspoon (5 mL) minced garlic
> 1 tablespoon (15 mL) olive oil
> 1 cup (236 mL) clam juice or reduced-fat chicken broth
> 3 tablespoons (21 g) chopped sun-dried tomatoes
> ¾ teaspoon (3.75 mL) each: dried marjoram and oregano leaves
> 1 can (8 ounces [240 mL]) reduced-sodium tomato sauce
> 4 halibut steaks (about 4 ounces [112 g] each)
> Salt and pepper, to taste

1. Sauté the onion and garlic in oil in a large skillet until browned, about 5 minutes. Stir in the clam juice, sun-dried tomatoes, marjoram, and oregano. Heat to boiling; boil, uncovered, stirring frequently until liquid is almost evaporated, about 5 minutes.

2. Add the tomato sauce and fish; simmer until the fish is tender and flakes with a fork, about 5 minutes. Season to taste with salt and pepper.

Per Serving: **Calories:** 204; **% of calories from fat:** 30; **Fat (g):** 6.8; **Saturated fat (g):** 0.9; **Cholesterol (mg):** 36.1; **Sodium (mg):** 232; **Protein (g):** 25.4; **Carbohydrate (g):** 9.6; **Exchanges:** Milk: 0.0; Vegetable: 2.0; Fruit: 0.0; Bread: 0.0; Meat: 3.0; Fat: 0.0

FLOUNDER EN PAPILLOTE

Traditionally made with a lean white fish, this recipe is also delicious with salmon or tuna.

6 SERVINGS

> 6 flounder, sole or other lean white fish fillets
>   (4 ounces each)
> Salt and pepper
> 1 cup each: sliced mushrooms (75 g), julienned carrots
>   (128 g)
> ¼ cup (38 g) finely chopped shallots or onion
> 2 cloves garlic, minced
> ½ teaspoon (2.5 mL) dried tarragon leaves
> 2 teaspoons (10 mL) margarine or butter
> ½ cup (118 mL) dry white wine or water
> ¼ cup (8 g) finely chopped parsley
> 6 lemon wedges

1. Cut six 12-inch (30-cm) squares of parchment paper; fold in half, and cut each into a large heart shape. Open the hearts and place 1 fish fillet on each; sprinkle lightly with salt and pepper.

2. Sauté the mushrooms, carrots, shallots, garlic, and tarragon in margarine in a large skillet until the carrots are crisp-tender, about 5 minutes. Stir in the wine and parsley; season to taste with salt and pepper. Spoon the mixture over fish. Fold the parchment paper in half, bringing edges together; crimp edges tightly to seal.

3. Bake on jelly-roll pan at 425°F (220°C) until packets puff, 10 to 12 minutes. Serve with lemon wedges.

Note: Foil can be used in place of parchment paper; bake fish 15 minutes.

Per Serving: **Calories: 149; % of calories from fat: 17; Fat (g): 2.8; Saturated fat (g): 0.6; Cholesterol (mg): 59.8; Sodium (mg): 118; Protein (g): 22.3; Carbohydrate (g): 5.7 Exchanges: Milk: 0.0; Vegetable: 1.0; Fruit: 0.0; Bread: 0.0; Meat: 2.5; Fat: 0.0**

HALIBUT WITH COUSCOUS

When preparing couscous, follow package directions, omitting salt and fat, and use either water or reduced-sodium chicken broth. Whole wheat couscous is available at natural foods stores. This recipe comes from Diabetes Snacks, Treats, and Easy Eats *by Barbara Grunes.*

6 (1-CUP [236-ML]) SERVINGS

> 1 cup each: flaked cooked halibut (150 g), grated carrot (110 g)
> 2 cups each: cooked couscous (314 g), baby spinach (360 g)
> ⅓ cup (16 g) chopped chives
> ¼ cup (59 mL) balsamic vinegar
> 1 tablespoon (15 mL) extra-virgin olive oil

1. Toss together the halibut, carrot, couscous, spinach, chives, vinegar, and oil.

Per Serving: **Calories: 121; % calories from fat: 22; Fat (g): 3; Saturated fat (g): 0.4; Cholesterol (mg): 7.7; Sodium (mg): 35; Protein (g): 7.6; Carbohydrate (g): 15.5 Exchanges: Milk: 0.0; Vegetable: 1.0; Fruit: 0.0; Bread: 0.5; Meat: 0.0; Fat: 1.0**

HALIBUT WITH SOUR CREAM AND POBLANO SAUCE >

The picante Sour Cream and Poblano Sauce is also excellent served with shredded chicken breast or lean pork in soft tacos, or over your favorite enchiladas.

4 SERVINGS

> 4 halibut steaks (about 4 ounces [112 g] each)
> 3 tablespoons (45 mL) lime juice
> 1 clove garlic, minced
> Salt and pepper, to taste
> Sour Cream and Poblano Sauce (recipe follows)
> 4 lime wedges

1. Brush the halibut with the combined lime juice and garlic; let stand 15 minutes. Cook the halibut in a lightly greased large skillet over medium heat until the halibut is tender and flakes with a fork, 4 to 5 minutes on each side. Season to taste with salt and pepper. Serve with Sour Cream and Poblano Sauce and lime wedges.

SOUR CREAM AND POBLANO SAUCE

ABOUT 1 CUP

> 1 each: thinly sliced large poblano chili pepper, finely chopped small onion
> 2 cloves garlic, minced
> 1 cup (236 mL) fat-free sour cream
> ¼ teaspoon (1.25 mL) ground cumin
> Salt and pepper, to taste

1. Sauté the chili pepper, onion, and garlic in a lightly greased small saucepan until very tender, about 5 minutes. Stir in the

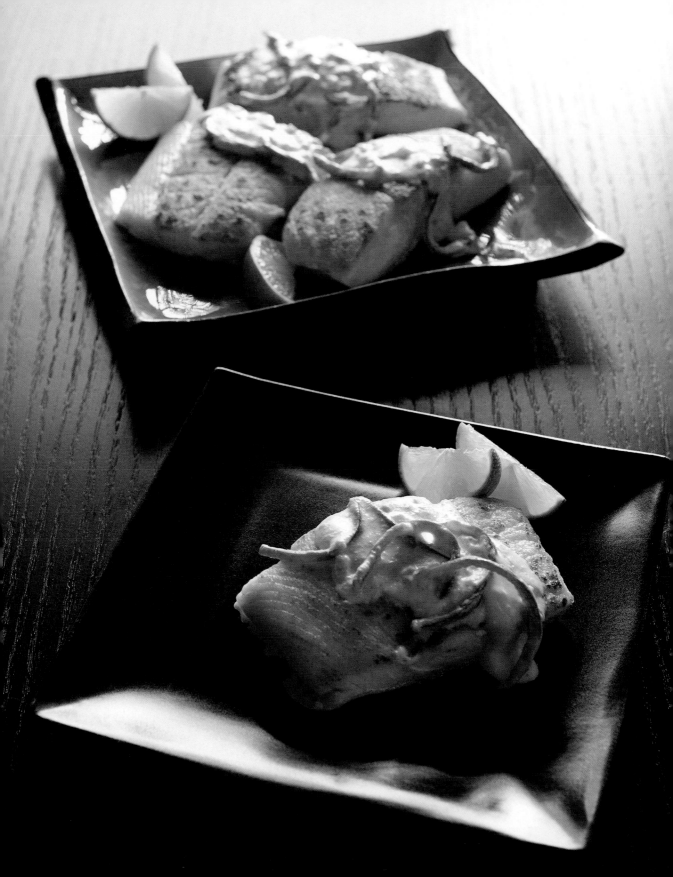

sour cream and cumin; cook over low heat 2 to 3 minutes. Season to taste with salt and pepper.

Per Serving: **Calories: 184; % of calories from fat: 13; Fat (g): 2.7; Saturated fat (g): 0.4; Cholesterol (mg): 36.4; Sodium (mg): 101; Protein (g): 28.2; Carbohydrate (g): 11.9 Exchanges: Milk: 0.0; Vegetable: 1.0; Fruit: 0.0; Bread: 0.0; Meat: 3.0; Fat: 0.0**

TERIYAKI SALMON BURGERS

Serve these burgers on their own or with all of the trimmings: whole wheat buns, lettuce, tomato, and pickle, as your eating plan allows.

4 BURGERS (1 BURGER PER SERVING)

> 8 ounces (224 g) skinless salmon fillet, cut into chunks
> ¼ cup (15 g) fresh bread crumbs
> 2 egg whites, slightly beaten
> 2 tablespoons (30 mL) each: reduced-sodium teriyaki sauce, dried onion flakes
> ¼ teaspoon (1.25 mL) pepper
> Butter-flavored cooking spray

1. Grind the salmon to a coarse texture by pulsing briefly in a food processor, or chop finely with a large, flat-bladed knife on a cutting board.

2. Combine the ground salmon, bread crumbs, egg whites, teriyaki sauce, onion flakes, and pepper in a bowl. Shape mixture into 4 burgers.

3. Lightly coat a nonstick skillet with cooking spray. Cook the burgers over medium heat until golden and cooked through, about 3 minutes on each side.

Per Serving: **Calories: 155; % calories from fat: 37; Fat (g): 6.3; Saturated fat (g): 1.5; Cholesterol (mg): 37.4; Sodium (mg): 332; Protein (g): 14.7; Carbohydrate (g): 9 Exchanges: Milk: 0.0; Vegetable: 0.0; Fruit: 0.0; Bread: 0.5; Meat: 2.0; Fat: 0.0**

RED SNAPPER BAKED WITH CILANTRO

Tuna, salmon, cod, or any firm white fish can be used in this recipe.

6 SERVINGS

⅓ cup (79 mL) lime juice
1½ tablespoons (22 mL) pickled jalapeño pepper juice
1 teaspoon (5 mL) ground cumin
1½ pounds (680 g) red snapper fillets or steaks
1 medium onion, thinly sliced
2 pickled jalapeño peppers, minced
2 cloves garlic, minced
1 cup (16 g) coarsely chopped cilantro
Salt and pepper, to taste
Thinly sliced green onions, for garnish
6 lime wedges

1. Pour combined lime juice, jalapeño juice, and cumin over fish in glass baking dish; top with onion, jalapeño peppers, garlic, and cilantro. Refrigerate, covered, 2 hours, turning fish once.

2. Bake uncovered, at 400°F (200°C) until red snapper is tender and flakes with a fork, about 10 minutes. Season to taste with salt and pepper; sprinkle with green onions and serve with lime wedges.

Per Serving: **Calories:** 135; **% of calories from fat:** 12; **Fat (g):** 1.7; **Saturated fat (g):** 0.3; **Cholesterol (mg):** 41.6; **Sodium (mg):** 169; **Protein (g):** 24; **Carbohydrate (g):** 5 Exchanges: **Milk:** 0.0; **Vegetable:** 0.0; **Fruit:** 0.0; **Bread:** 0.0; **Meat:** 3.0; **Fat:** 0.0

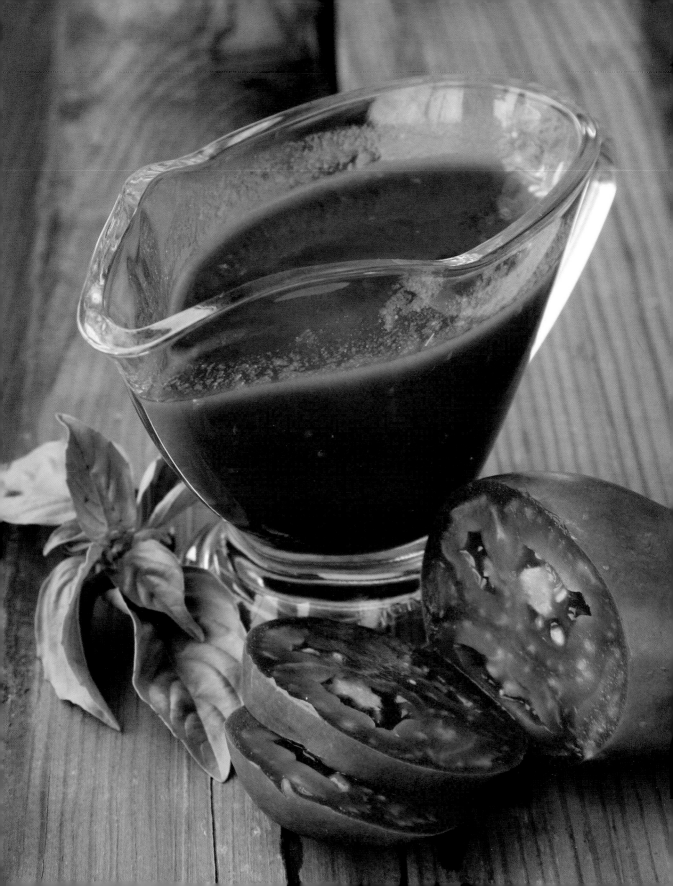

SAUCES

10-MINUTE SPAGHETTI SAUCE

Cooking tomatoes releases an important nutrient called lycopene, which is thought to have significant heart-protective health benefits. Keep cooked tomato sauce on hand in the refrigerator or freezer to use on pasta and in casseroles, as a dipper with cut-up vegetables, and as a pizza topper or bread spread.

8 (1-CUP [236-ML]) SERVINGS

> Olive oil cooking spray
>
> 1 cup each: chopped onion (150 g), zucchini (124 g), grated carrots (110 g)
>
> 1 can (28 ounces [794 g]) reduced-sodium crushed tomatoes, undrained
>
> 2 cans (8 ounces [224 mL] each) reduced-sodium tomato sauce
>
> 1 tablespoon (15 mL) Italian seasoning

1. Lightly coat a nonstick saucepan with cooking spray. Heat over medium heat. Add the onion, zucchini, and carrots and cook, partially covered and stirring occasionally, for 5 minutes or until tender.

2. Stir in the tomatoes with juice, tomato sauce, and seasoning. Heat to boiling. Reduce heat to a brisk simmer and cook, uncovered, for 5 minutes.

Per Serving: **Calories:** 51; **% calories from fat:** 5; **Fat (g):** 0.3; **Saturated fat (g):** 0; **Cholesterol (mg):** 0; **Sodium (mg):** 43; **Protein (g):** 2.3; **Carbohydrate (g):** 9.7 Exchanges: **Milk:** 0.0; **Vegetable:** 2.0; **Fruit:** 0.0; **Bread:** 0.0; **Meat:** 0.0; **Fat:** 0.0

RUSTIC TOMATO SAUCE

This is another sauce that does double duty as a pasta or pizza topper. Try it over steamed vegetables for a change of pace.

ABOUT 14 (¼-CUP [59-ML]) SERVINGS

> Olive oil cooking spray
> ¼ cup (59 mL) water
> 4 cloves garlic, minced
> 1¼ cups (188 g) chopped onions
> 1 can (28 ounces [794 g]) reduced-sodium plum
>   tomatoes, undrained
> 1 can (6 ounces [170 g]) reduced-sodium tomato paste
> 2 teaspoons (10 mL) ground oregano

1. Lightly coat a large nonstick saucepan with cooking spray and warm the pan over medium heat. Add the water, garlic, onions, and tomatoes. Cook 2 minutes. Stir in the tomato paste and oregano.

2. Heat the sauce to boiling. Reduce the heat to medium-low and simmer uncovered for 25 minutes, stirring occasionally. The sauce will thicken as it cooks. Remove from heat. Use immediately or cool and refrigerate.

Tip: For a chunkier sauce, add ½ cup diced celery.

Per Serving: **Calories: 28; % calories from fat: 5; Fat (g): 0.2; Saturated fat (g): 0; Cholesterol (mg): 0; Sodium (mg): 17; Protein (g): 1.2; Carbohydrate (g): 6.5 Exchanges: Milk: 0.0; Vegetable: 1.0; Fruit: 0.0; Bread: 0.0; Meat: 0.0; Fat: 0.0**

BARBECUE SAUCE

Traditional barbecue sauce is high in carbohydrates and sodium, making it unsuitable for most eating plans. Our version lightens up considerably, thanks to spoonable brown sugar substitute. If your supermarket does not carry brown sugar substitute, use a spoonable granulated sugar substitute or sugar-free maple-flavored syrup. If using syrup, cook the sauce a little longer to desired thickness.

8 SERVINGS (2 TABLESPOONS [30 ML] PER SERVING)

> Butter-flavored cooking spray
> ½ cup each: chopped onion (150 g), green bell pepper
>   (150 g), water (120 mL)
> ⅓ cup (79 mL) ketchup
> 1 teaspoon (5 mL) barbecue spice mix
> 2½ tablespoons (38 mL) red wine vinegar
> 2 teaspoons (10 mL) Worcestershire sauce
> 3 tablespoons (42 g) spoonable brown sugar substitute

1. Lightly coat a saucepan with cooking spray. Cook the onion and bell pepper over medium heat, stirring occasionally, 5 minutes or until tender.

2. Stir in the water, ketchup, spice mix, vinegar, Worcestershire sauce, and sugar substitute. Simmer for 5 minutes.

3. Spoon the sauce into covered container and store in refrigerator. Stir before serving.

Per Serving: **Calories: 20; % calories from fat: 3; Fat (g): 0.1; Saturated fat (g):** 0; **Cholesterol (mg): 0; Sodium (mg): 126; Protein (g): 0.4; Carbohydrate (g): 5** Exchanges: **Milk: 0.0; Vegetable: 0.0; Fruit: 0.0; Bread: 0.0; Meat: 0.0; Fat: 0.0**

THAI PEANUT SAUCE

This sauce is traditionally made with coconut milk, which is high in fat. We've reduced the fat by using evaporated skim milk and reduced-fat peanut butter. The sauce can also be used as a dipper for vegetables and as a topper for rice dishes. Spice it up, if you wish, with a dash of cayenne pepper or hot sauce. This recipe comes from Diabetes Snacks, Treats, and Easy Eats *by Barbara Grunes.*

8 SERVINGS (2 TABLESPOONS [30 ML] PER SERVING)

½ cup (118 mL) evaporated skim milk (not condensed)

¼ cup each: reduced-fat peanut butter (65 g), chopped onion (38 g)

1 teaspoon (5 mL) each: lemon juice, chopped gingerroot or ground ginger

1.   Whisk together the milk, peanut butter, onion, lemon juice, and gingerroot in saucepan. Simmer the mixture a few minutes until smooth and heated through.

2.   Serve hot or pour into a container and refrigerate covered until ready to serve.

Serving Suggestion: Dress up the sauce for company with a garnish of chopped peanuts and cilantro leaves.

Per Serving: **Calories: 62**; **% calories from fat: 42**; **Fat (g): 3**; **Saturated fat (g): 0.6**; **Cholesterol (mg): 0.6**; **Sodium (mg): 81**; **Protein (g): 3.3**; **Carbohydrate (g): 6.1** Exchanges: **Milk: 0.0**; **Vegetable: 0.0**; **Fruit: 0.0**; **Bread: 0.5**; **Meat: 0.0**; **Fat: 0.5**

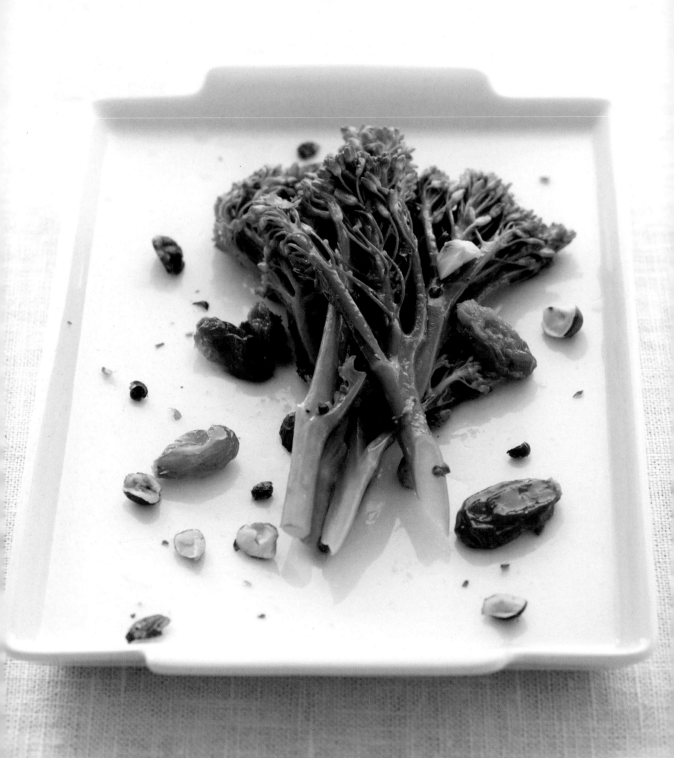

SIDE DISHES

BROCCOLI RABE SAUTÉED WITH GARLIC

This simple, flavorful vegetable recipe can also be made with broccoli, green beans, or asparagus.

4–6 SERVINGS

> 1 pound (454 g) broccoli rabe, cooked crisp-tender
> 4 cloves garlic, minced
> Salt and pepper, to taste

1. Sauté the broccoli rabe and garlic in a lightly greased large skillet until the broccoli rabe is beginning to brown, 4 to 5 minutes. Season to taste with salt and pepper.

Per Serving: **Calories:** 32; **% of calories from fat:** 8; **Fat (g):** 0.4; **Saturated fat (g):** 0.1; **Cholesterol (mg):** 0; **Sodium (mg):** 25; **Protein (g):** 3.1; **Carbohydrate (g):** 5.9 Exchanges: **Milk:** 0.0; **Vegetable:** 1.0; **Fruit:** 0.0; **Bread:** 0.0; **Meat:** 0.0; **Fat:** 0.0

CAULIFLOWER WITH CREAMY CHEESE SAUCE

For flavor variations, make the cheese sauce with other reduced-fat cheeses, such as Havarti, Gruyère, American, or blue.

6 SERVINGS

> 1 large head cauliflower (about 2 pounds [908 g]), sliced
> Creamy Cheese Sauce (recipe follows)
> Paprika, for garnish

1. Cook the cauliflower in 2 inches (5 cm) of simmering water in a medium saucepan, covered, until tender, 20 to 25 minutes; drain. Spoon Creamy Cheese Sauce over and sprinkle with paprika.

CREAMY CHEESE SAUCE

ABOUT 1¼ CUPS (295 ML)

> 2 tablespoons (30 mL) minced onion
> 1 tablespoon (15 mL) margarine or butter
> 2 tablespoons (30 mL) all-purpose flour
> 1 cup (236 mL) fat-free milk
> ½ cup (2 ounces [56 g]) cubed reduced-fat pasteurized processed cheese
> ¼ teaspoon (1.25 mL) dry mustard
> 2–3 drops red pepper sauce
> Salt and white pepper, to taste

1. Sauté the onion in margarine in a small saucepan 2 to 3 minutes. Stir in the flour; cook 1 minute. Whisk in the milk and heat to boiling; boil, stirring until thickened, about 1 minute. Reduce heat to low; add the cheese, mustard, and pepper sauce, whisking until the cheese is melted. Season to taste with salt and white pepper.

Per Serving: **Calories:** 102; **% of calories from fat:** 31; **Fat (g):** 3.6; **Saturated fat (g):** 1.5; **Cholesterol (mg):** 5.7; **Sodium (mg):** 194; **Protein (g):** 6.5; **Carbohydrate (g):** 11.7 Exchanges: **Milk:** 0.0; **Vegetable:** 2.0; **Fruit:** 0.0; **Bread:** 0.0; **Meat:** 0.5; **Fat:** 0.5

GREEK-STYLE GREEN BEANS

Fresh green beans are long simmered with tomatoes, herbs, and garlic in traditional Greek style.

4–6 SERVINGS

½ cup (75 g) chopped onion

4 cloves garlic, minced

¾ teaspoon (3.75 mL) each: dried oregano and basil leaves

1 tablespoon (15 mL) olive oil

1 can (28 ounces [794 g]) reduced-sodium tomatoes, undrained, coarsely chopped

1 pound (454 g) green beans

Salt and pepper, to taste

1. Sauté the onion, garlic, oregano, and basil in oil in a large skillet until onion is tender, 3 to 4 minutes. Add the tomatoes with liquid and green beans and heat to boiling; reduce heat and simmer, covered, until the beans are very tender, about 30 minutes. Season to taste with salt and pepper.

Per Serving: **Calories:** 123; **% of calories from fat:** 28; **Fat (g):** 4.3; **Saturated fat (g):** 0.6; **Cholesterol (mg):** 0; **Sodium (mg):** 30; **Protein (g):** 4.5; **Carbohydrate (g):** 20.5 Exchanges: **Milk:** 0.0; **Vegetable:** 4.0; **Fruit:** 0.0; **Bread:** 0.0; **Meat:** 0.0; **Fat:** 0.5

ASPARAGUS WITH LEMON–WINE SAUCE

This rich sauce is also delicious served with crisp-tender broccoli, cauliflower, green beans, or Brussels sprouts. This recipe comes from 1,001 Delicious Recipes for People with Diabetes by Sue Spitler.

4 SERVINGS

> 2 tablespoons (30 mL) minced shallots or green onions
> ¼ cup (59 mL) dry white wine or water
> ¾ cup (59 mL) fat-free half-and-half or milk
> 1 tablespoon (15 mL) all-purpose flour
> ½ teaspoon (2.5 mL) each: dried thyme and marjoram leaves
> 1 tablespoon (15 mL) lemon juice
> Salt and white pepper, to taste
> 1 pound (454 g) asparagus spears, cooked crisp-tender, warm

1. Sauté the shallots in a lightly greased small saucepan until tender, 2 to 3 minutes. Add the wine and heat to boiling; reduce heat and simmer, uncovered, until wine is evaporated, 3 to 4 minutes. Stir in the combined half-and-half, flour, thyme, and marjoram; heat to boiling. Boil, stirring until thickened, about 1 minute. Stir in the lemon juice; season to taste with salt and pepper. Spoon over asparagus.

Per Serving: **Calories:** 85; **% of calories from fat:** 4; **Fat (g):** 0.4; **Saturated fat (g):** 0.1; **Cholesterol (mg):** 0; **Sodium (mg):** 59; **Protein (g):** 4.8; **Carbohydrate (g):** 13.4 Exchanges: **Milk:** 0.0; **Vegetable:** 2.0; **Fruit:** 0.0; **Bread:** 0.5; **Meat:** 0.0; **Fat:** 0.0

MUSHROOMS WITH SOUR CREAM >

Cooking the mushrooms very slowly until deeply browned intensifies their flavor. Especially delicious served with pierogi, ravioli, or grilled eggplant slices.

4 SERVINGS

12 ounces (340 g) shiitake or cremini mushrooms, stems discarded, sliced

¼ cup (38 g) finely chopped onion

1 teaspoon (5 mL) minced garlic

¼ cup (59 mL) dry white wine or reduced-sodium vegetable broth

¼ teaspoon (1.25 mL) dried thyme leaves

½ cup (118 mL) fat-free sour cream

Salt and cayenne pepper, to taste

1. Sauté the mushrooms, onion, and garlic in a lightly greased large skillet 3 to 4 minutes. Add the wine and thyme; heat to boiling. Reduce heat and simmer, covered, until the mushrooms are tender, 8 to 10 minutes. Cook, uncovered, on low heat until the mushrooms are dry and well browned, about 20 to 25 minutes. Stir in the sour cream; season to taste with salt and cayenne pepper.

Per Serving: Calories: 80; % of calories from fat: 2; Fat (g): 0.2; Saturated fat (g): 0.1; Cholesterol (mg): 0; Sodium (mg): 24; Protein (g): 3.5; Carbohydrate (g): 16.5 Exchanges: Milk: 0.0; Vegetable: 2.0; Fruit: 0.0; Bread: 0.5; Meat: 0.0; Fat: 0.0

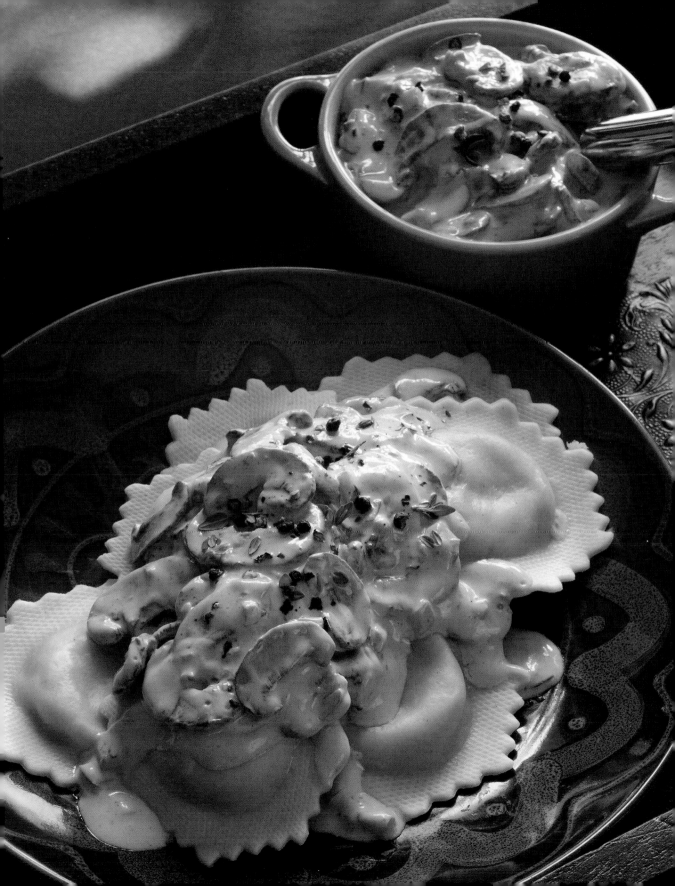

HONEY-GLAZED ROASTED BEETS

Roasting maximizes the sweet flavor of beets.

6 SERVINGS

> 1½ pounds (680 g) medium beets
> Vegetable oil cooking spray
> 2 medium red onions, cut into wedges
> ¼ cup (41 g) currants or raisins
> 3–4 tablespoons (19–25 g) toasted walnuts
> ¼ cup (59 mL) honey
> 2–3 tablespoons (30–45 mL) red wine vinegar
> 1 tablespoon (15 mL) canola oil
> 4 cloves garlic, minced
> Salt and pepper, to taste

1. Arrange the beets and onions in a single layer on a greased foil-lined jelly-roll pan; spray with cooking spray. Roast at 425°F (220°C) until beets are tender, about 40 minutes.

2. Peel the beets and cut into 1-inch (2.5-cm) pieces. Combine the beets, onions, currants, and walnuts; heat the combined remaining ingredients, except salt and pepper, pour over the vegetables and toss. Season to taste with salt and pepper.

Per Serving: **Calories: 94; % of calories from fat: 18; Fat (g): 1.9; Saturated fat (g): 0.4; Cholesterol (mg): 0; Sodium (mg): 70; Protein (g): 1.1; Carbohydrate (g): 19.3** Exchanges: **Milk: 0.0; Vegetable: 2.0; Fruit: 0.0; Bread: 0.5; Meat: 0.0; Fat: 0.0**

EGGPLANT AND VEGETABLE SAUTÉ

Minced roasted garlic is available in jars in your produce section; substitute fresh minced garlic if desired.

6 SERVINGS

> 1 large eggplant (about 1¼ pounds [566 g]), unpeeled, cubed
>
> 3 cups (450 g) frozen stir-fry pepper blend
>
> 4 teaspoons (20 mL) minced roasted garlic
>
> ½ teaspoon (2.5 mL) each: dried rosemary and thyme leaves
>
> 2 teaspoons (10 mL) olive oil
>
> 1 can (15 ounces [425 g]) cannellini or Great Northern beans, rinsed, drained
>
> Salt and pepper, to taste

1. Cook the eggplant, pepper blend, garlic, rosemary, and thyme in oil in a large saucepan over medium heat, covered, until the vegetables are tender, 8 to 10 minutes; stir in the beans and cook until hot, about 2 minutes. Season to taste with salt and pepper.

Per Serving: **Calories:** 109; **% of calories from fat:** 16; **Fat (g):** 2; **Saturated fat (g):** 0.3; **Cholesterol (mg):** 0; **Sodium (mg):** 114; **Protein (g):** 4.1; **Carbohydrate (g):** 19.1 Exchanges: **Milk:** 0.0; **Vegetable:** 2.0; **Fruit:** 0.0; **Bread:** 1.0; **Meat:** 0.0; **Fat:** 0.5

FRIED BROWN RICE

Brown rice is a good nutritional choice because it is rich in magnesium, phosphorus, and selenium and has vitamin B6, dietary fiber, thiamin, and niacin. Brown rice takes longer to cook than white rice, but instant brown rice takes only 10 minutes. This recipe comes from Diabetes Snacks, Treats, and Easy Eats *by Barbara Grunes.*

8 (1-CUP [236-ML]) SERVINGS

> Canola oil cooking spray
> ½ cup each: chopped onion (75 g), grated carrot (45 g)
> 3 cups (480 g) cooked brown rice
> 2 cups (208 g) fresh bean sprouts, rinsed, drained
> 1 package (10 ounces [280 g]) frozen green peas, thawed
> 3 tablespoons (45 mL) soy sauce

1. Lightly coat a nonstick skillet or wok with cooking spray.

2. Cook the onions over medium heat, stirring constantly, until tender, about 5 minutes. Lightly spray the pan again. Add the carrot, rice, bean sprouts, peas, and soy sauce. Cook, stirring constantly, until hot, about 2 minutes.

Serving Suggestion: For a hearty main dish, add 1 lightly beaten egg and/or 1 cup diced tofu when cooking the rice and vegetable mixture.

Per Serving: **Calories: 127;** % calories from fat: 6; Fat (g): 0.8; Saturated fat (g): 0.2; Cholesterol (mg): 0; Sodium (mg): 425; Protein (g): 5; Carbohydrate (g): 25.5 Exchanges: **Milk: 0.0; Vegetable: 0.0; Fruit: 0.0; Bread: 2.0; Meat: 0.0; Fat: 0.0**

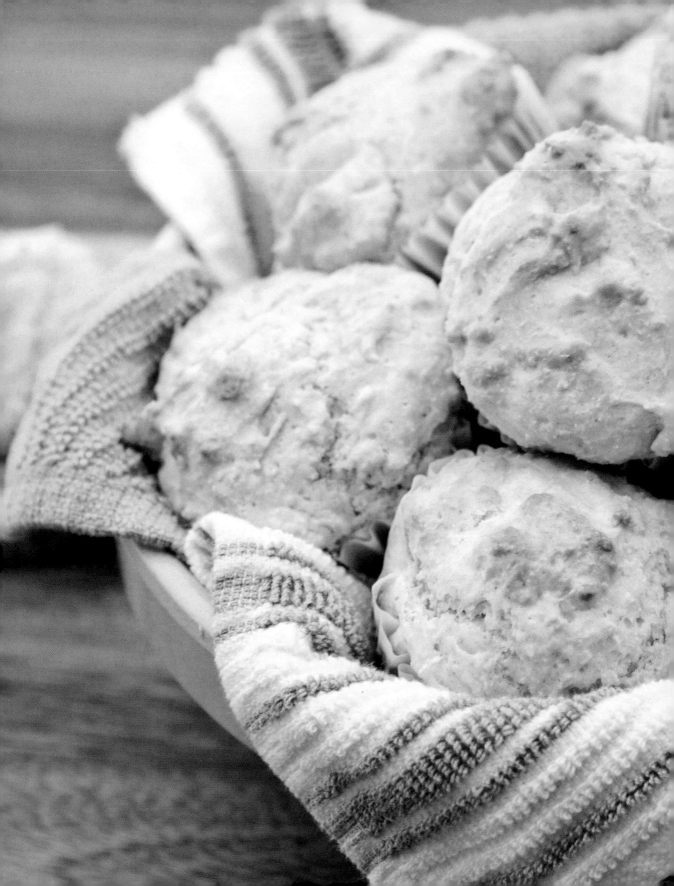

BREADS

CHEDDAR BISCUITS

Lighter-than-air biscuits require a light touch when it comes to mixing. If using your fingertips to cut the margarine into the flour, work quickly and lightly. A light touch also helps when stirring the yogurt and cheese into the flour mixture.

18 BISCUITS (1 BISCUIT PER SERVING)

Butter-flavored cooking spray
½ cup (112 g) margarine
2 cups (242 g) self-rising flour (see note)
1¼ cups (295 mL) nonfat plain yogurt
1 cup (4 ounces [112 g]) shredded reduced-fat mild Cheddar cheese

1. Preheat oven to 450°F (240°C). Lightly coat a nonstick baking sheet with cooking spray.

2. Cut the margarine into the flour using a pastry blender, 2 knives, or fingertips until the mixture is crumbly. Stir in the yogurt and cheese, mixing lightly just until ingredients are combined.

3. Drop batter by the tablespoonful onto baking sheet. Bake 10 to 12 minutes or until biscuits are golden.

Note: If self-rising flour is not available where you shop, make your own by adding 1 tablespoon (15 mL) of salt and 5 tablespoons (74 g) of baking powder to every 8 cups (968 g) of all-purpose flour.

Per Serving: **Calories: 128; % calories from fat: 50; Fat (g): 6.8; Saturated fat (g): 2.3; Cholesterol (mg): 4.8; Sodium (mg): 243; Protein (g): 3.9; Carbohydrate (g): 11.7** Exchanges: **Milk: 0.0; Vegetable: 0.0; Fruit: 0.0; Bread: 1.0; Meat: 0.0; Fat: 1.0**

CORN BREAD

If you prefer corn muffins, just spray a muffin pan with 2½-inch cups. Pour in batter until half full. Bake 25 to 30 minutes and serve hot.

16 SERVINGS (EACH SERVING A 2-INCH [5-CM] SQUARE)

> **Butter-flavored cooking spray**
> **1 cup (121 g) all-purpose flour**
> **1 cup (160 g) yellow cornmeal**
> **½ teaspoon (2.5 mL) baking soda**
> **2 teaspoons (10 mL) baking powder**
> **1 egg, beaten**
> **1 cup (236 mL) low-fat buttermilk**
> **3 tablespoons (42 g) margarine, melted**

1. Preheat oven to 425°F (220°C). Spray an 8 × 8-inch (20 cm × 20-cm) pan.

2. Sift together flour, cornmeal, baking soda, and powder in a large bowl. Combine egg, buttermilk, and margarine. Add to flour mixture, stirring well to combine ingredients. Do not overmix.

3. Pour the batter into the prepared pan. Bake in the center of the oven 20 to 25 minutes. Cool Corn Bread slightly. Cut into 16 (2-inch [5-cm]) squares. Serve warm.

Per Serving: **Calories: 85.9; % calories from fat: 30.4; Fat (g): 2.9; Saturated fat (g): 0.6; Cholesterol (mg): 13.8; Sodium (mg): 148.5; Protein (g): 2.3; Carbohydrate (g): 12.7** Exchanges: **Milk: 0.0; Vegetable: 0.0; Fruit: 0.0; Bread: 1.0; Meat: 0.0; Fat: 0.5**

SQUASH DINNER ROLLS >

Use pumpkin, Hubbard, or acorn squash for these rolls; mashed sweet potatoes can be used also. If a loaf is preferred, bake in a greased 8 × 4-inch (20 × 10-cm) loaf pan until the loaf is browned and sounds hollow when tapped, about 40 minutes.

24 ROLLS (1 EACH)

1½–2½ cups (182–303 g) all-purpose flour, divided
1 cup (135 g) whole wheat flour
2 packages fast-rising yeast
1–2 teaspoons (5–10 mL) salt
½ cup (118 mL) fat-free milk
¼ cup (59 mL) honey
1–2 tablespoons (15–30 mL) margarine or butter
¾ cup (184 g) mashed cooked winter squash
1 egg

1. Combine 1½ cups (182 g) all-purpose flour, whole wheat flour, yeast, and salt in large bowl. Heat the milk, honey, and margarine in a small saucepan to 125–130°F (52–54°C); add to the flour mixture, mixing until smooth. Mix in the squash, egg, and enough of the remaining 1 cup (121 g) all-purpose flour to make a smooth dough.

2. Knead the dough on a floured surface until smooth and elastic, about 5 minutes. Place in a greased bowl; let stand, covered, in a warm place until double in size, 30 to 45 minutes. Punch dough down.

3. Preheat oven to 375°F (190°C). Grease muffin pans (24 cups).

4. Divide the dough into 24 pieces; shape into round rolls and place in muffin cups or on an unlined baking sheet. Bake until browned, 20 to 25 minutes.

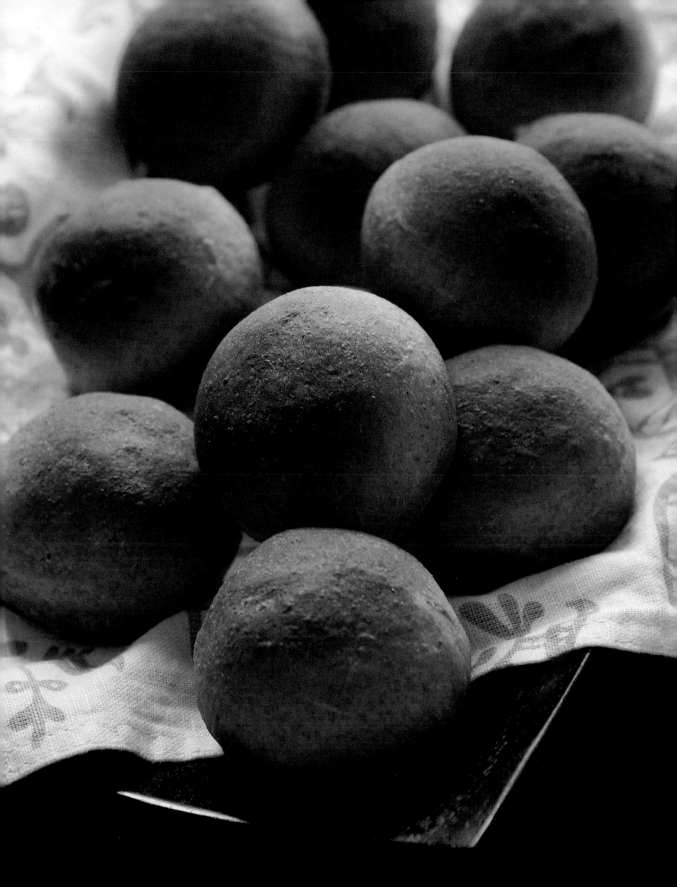

VARIATION

Raisin-Walnut Pumpkin Bread—Make recipe as above, substituting mashed cooked or canned pumpkin for the squash and adding ½ cup each raisins (83 g) and chopped walnuts (57 g). Shape into a loaf in 9 × 5-inch (22.5 × 13-cm) loaf pan and let rise; bake at 375°F (190°C) until the loaf is browned and sounds hollow when tapped, about 40 minutes.

Per Serving: Calories: 70; % of calories from fat: 11; Fat (g): 0.9; Saturated fat (g): 0.2; Cholesterol (mg): 9; Sodium (mg): 100; Protein (g): 2.2; Carbohydrate (g): 13.5 Exchanges: Milk: 0.0; Vegetable: 0.0; Fruit: 0.0; Bread: 1.0; Meat: 0.0; Fat: 0.0

ROASTED RED PEPPER BREAD

Bake this loaf in a freeform long or round shape, or in a pan. For convenience, use jarred roasted red pepper.

1 LOAF (16 SERVINGS)

> 2¼–2¾ cups (272 g–333 g) all-purpose flour, divided
> ¾ cup (101 g) whole wheat flour
> ¼ cup (23 g) grated fat-free Parmesan cheese
> 1½ teaspoons (7.5 mL) dried Italian seasoning, divided
> ½ teaspoon (2.5 mL) salt
> 1 package fast-rising active dry yeast
> 1¼ cups (295 mL) very hot water (125–130°F [52–54°C])
> 1 tablespoon (15 mL) olive oil
> 4 ounces (112 g) reduced-fat mozzarella cheese, cubed (½ inch [1 cm])
> ½ cup (75 g) coarsely chopped roasted red pepper
> 1 egg white, beaten

1. Combine 2¼ cups (272 g) all-purpose flour, whole wheat flour, Parmesan cheese, 1 teaspoon (5 mL) Italian seasoning, salt, and yeast in a large bowl; add hot water and oil, mixing until blended. Mix in the mozzarella cheese, red pepper, and enough remaining ½ cup (61 g) all-purpose flour to make a smooth dough.

2. Knead the dough on a floured surface until smooth and elastic, about 5 minutes. Place in a greased bowl; let rise, covered, in a warm place until double in size, about 30 minutes. Punch dough down.

3. Shape dough into loaf and place in greased 9 × 5-inch (22.5 cm × 13-cm) loaf pan. Let stand, covered, until double in size, about 30 minutes.

4. Preheat oven to 375°F (190°C).

5. Make 3 or 4 slits in top of the loaf with a sharp knife. Brush egg white over dough and sprinkle with the remaining Italian seasoning. Bake until the loaf is golden and sounds hollow when tapped, 35 to 40 minutes. Remove from pan and cool on wire rack.

Per Serving: **Calories: 119**; **% of calories from fat: 16**; **Fat (g): 2.2**; **Saturated fat (g): 0.9**; **Cholesterol (mg): 3.8**; **Sodium (mg): 133**; **Protein (g): 5.6**; **Carbohydrate (g): 19** Exchanges: **Milk: 0.0**; **Vegetable: 0.0**; **Fruit: 0.0**; **Bread: 1.5**; **Meat: 0.0**; **Fat: 0.5**

BANANA BREAD

Brown sugar gives this banana bread a caramel flavor; the applesauce adds moistness. It's the best!

1 LOAF (16 SERVINGS)

4 tablespoons (57 g) margarine or butter, room temperature

¼ cup (59 mL) applesauce

2 eggs

2 tablespoons (30 mL) fat-free milk or water

¾ cup (169 g) packed light brown sugar

1 cup (225 g) mashed banana (2–3 medium bananas)

1¾ cups (212 g) all-purpose flour

2 teaspoons (10 mL) baking powder

½ teaspoon (2.5 mL) baking soda

¼ teaspoon (1.25 mL) salt

¼ cup (29 g) coarsely chopped walnuts or pecans

1. Preheat oven to 350°F (180°C). Grease a 8 × 4-inch (20 cm × 10-cm) loaf pan.

2. Beat the margarine, applesauce, eggs, milk, and brown sugar in a large mixer bowl until smooth. Add the banana and mix at low speed; beat at high speed 1 to 2 minutes. Mix in the combined flour, baking powder, baking soda, and salt; mix in walnuts. Pour into prepared loaf pan. Bake until bread is golden and a toothpick inserted into center comes out clean, 55 to 60 minutes. Cool in pan 10 minutes; remove from pan and cool on wire rack.

Per Serving: **Calories:** 151; **% of calories from fat:** 28; **Fat (g):** 4.8; **Saturated fat (g):** 0.9; **Cholesterol (mg):** 26.7; **Sodium (mg):** 160; **Protein (g):** 2.9; **Carbohydrate (g):** 24.9 Exchanges: **Milk:** 0.0; **Vegetable:** 0.0; **Fruit:** 0.5; **Bread:** 1.0; **Meat:** 0.0; **Fat:** 1.0

MULTIGRAIN BATTER BREAD

Batter bread preparation is quick and easy, requiring no kneading and only one rise.

2 LOAVES (16 SERVINGS EACH)

3¼ cups (393 g) all-purpose flour
1 cup (135 g) whole wheat flour
¼ cup (23 g) soy flour or quick-cooking oats
¾ cup (68 g) quick-cooking oats
¼ cup (50 g) sugar
½ teaspoon (2.5 mL) salt
2 packages fast-rising yeast
1 cup (160 g) cooked brown rice
2¼ cups (532 mL) fat-free milk, hot (125–130°F [52–54°C])
2 tablespoons (30 mL) vegetable oil

1. Grease two 8 × 4-inch (20 cm × 10-cm) loaf pans.

2. Combine the flours, oats, sugar, salt, and yeast in a large bowl; add the rice, milk, and oil, mixing until smooth. Spoon into prepared loaf pans; let stand, covered, until double in size, about 30 minutes.

3. Preheat oven to 375°F (190°C). Bake until the loaves are browned and sound hollow when tapped, 35 to 40 minutes. Remove from pans and cool on wire racks.

Per Serving: **Calories:** 97; **% of calories from fat:** 13; **Fat (g):** 1.4; **Saturated fat (g):** 0.2; **Cholesterol (mg):** 0.3; **Sodium (mg):** 43; **Protein (g):** 3.5; **Carbohydrate (g):** 17.9 Exchanges: **Milk:** 0.0; **Vegetable:** 0.0; **Fruit:** 0.0; **Bread:** 1.0; **Meat:** 0.0; **Fat:** 0.5

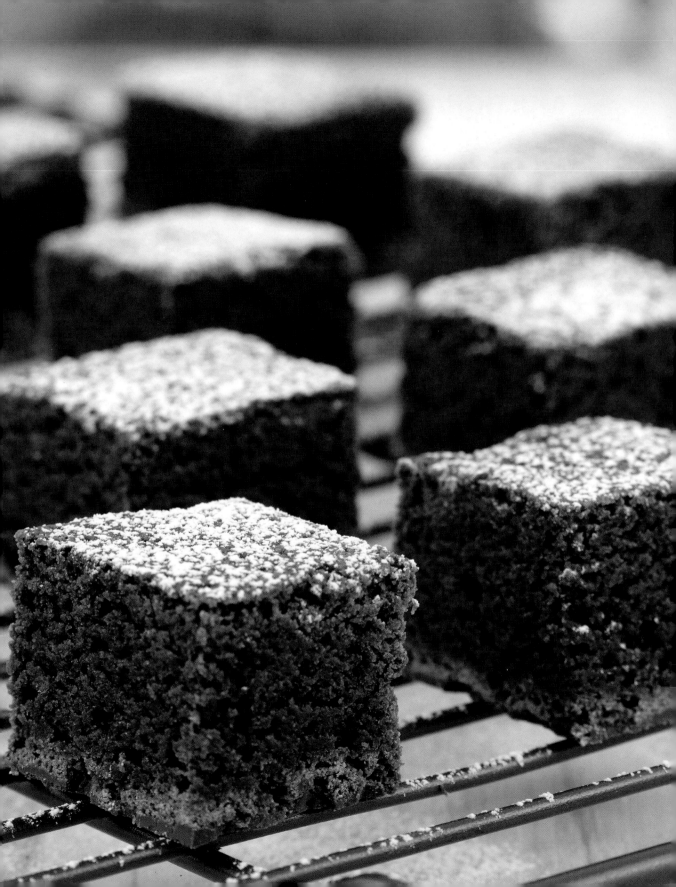

DESSERTS

BEST BROWNIES

It's possible to still enjoy rich, chewy brownies as long as you keep the serving size reasonable.

16 BROWNIES (1 BROWNIE PER SERVING)

> Butter-flavored cooking spray
> ⅓ cup (75 g) reduced-fat margarine, melted and slightly cooled
> ⅓ cup (29 g) cocoa powder
> ½ cup (118 mL) egg substitute
> ¾ cup (80 g) cake flour
> ½ cup (100 g) sugar
> ½ teaspoon (2.5 mL) baking powder
> 1½ (7.5 mL) teaspoons vanilla
> Confectioners' sugar, for dusting

1. Position the oven rack in center and preheat oven to 350°F (180°C). Lightly coat an 8-inch (20-cm) square nonstick baking pan with cooking spray.

2. Whisk together the margarine and cocoa in bowl. Blend in the egg substitute.

3. Sift together the flour, sugar, and baking powder in large bowl. Stir margarine mixture into flour mixture. Add vanilla.

4. Pour the batter into the prepared pan. Bake until a cake tester or toothpick inserted into center comes out dry and clean, 25 minutes.

5. Cool the brownies in pan. Cut into squares. Rest on rack and dust with confectioners' sugar.

Per Serving: **Calories:** 67; **% calories from fat:** 27; **Fat (g):** 2.1; **Saturated fat (g):** 0.4; **Cholesterol (mg):** 0; **Sodium (mg):** 75; **Protein (g):** 1.5; **Carbohydrate (g):** 11.2
Exchanges: **Milk:** 0.0; **Vegetable:** 0.0; **Fruit:** 0.0; **Bread:** 1.0; **Meat:** 0.0; **Fat:** 0.0

STRAWBERRY SHORTCAKE

With store-bought angel food cake, this dessert is a breeze to make as well as lower in fat and calories than the traditional dessert.

4 SERVINGS (1 SLICE PER SERVING)

> 4 slices angel food cake, store-bought or homemade
> 1 cup (236 mL) sugar-free nondairy whipped topping
> 3 cups (498 g) sliced strawberries
> 2 tablespoons (30 mL) sugar or sugar substitute

1. Arrange a slice of angel food cake on each plate. Spoon whipped topping onto cake and sprinkle with strawberries and sugar.

Per Serving: **Calories:** 168; **% calories from fat:** 13; **Fat (g):** 2.5; **Saturated fat (g):** 1; **Cholesterol (mg):** 0; **Sodium (mg):** 61; **Protein (g):** 4.4; **Carbohydrate (g):** 31.4 Exchanges: **Milk:** 0.0; **Vegetable:** 0.0; **Fruit:** 1.0; **Bread:** 1.0; **Meat:** 0.0; **Fat:** 0.5

STRAWBERRY CREAM PIE >

Celebrate spring with this colorful fresh berry pie.

8 SERVINGS

1¼ cups (125 g) reduced-fat graham cracker crumbs
4–5 tablespoons (57–71 g) margarine or butter, melted
6¼ teaspoons (22 g) Equal® for Recipes or 19 packets
   Equal® sweetener, divided
8 ounces (224 g) fat-free cream cheese, room temperature
1 teaspoon (5 mL) boiling water
1 package (0.3 ounces [8 g]) sugar-free strawberry gelatin
2 cups (332 g) sliced strawberries
Light whipped topping, as garnish

1. Preheat oven to 350°F (180°C).

2. Mix the graham cracker crumbs, margarine, and 1 teaspoon (5 mL) Equal® for Recipes in 8-inch (20-cm) pie pan;
   pat evenly on bottom and side of pan. Bake until lightly
   browned, 6 to 8 minutes. Cool.

3. Beat the cream cheese, vanilla, and 1¾ teaspoons (8.75 mL)
   Equal® for Recipes in a small bowl until fluffy; spread evenly
   in bottom of crust.

4. Pour boiling water over gelatin and remaining 3½ (17.5 mL)
   teaspoons Equal® for Recipes in bowl, whisking until gelatin is dissolved. Refrigerate until mixture is the consistency
   of unbeaten egg whites, 20 to 30 minutes. Arrange half the
   strawberries over the cream cheese; spoon half the gelatin
   mixture over the strawberries. Arrange the remaining strawberries over the pie and spoon the remaining gelatin mixture
   over.

5. Refrigerate until the pie is set and chilled, 2 to 3 hours. Serve
   with light whipped topping.

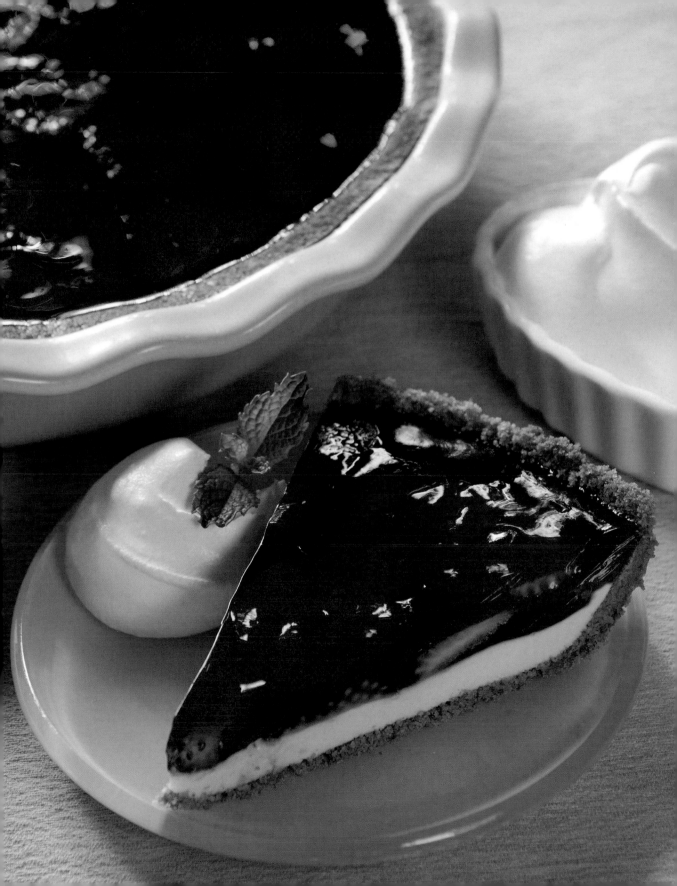

VARIATIONS

Double Berry Pie—Make recipe as above, substituting 1 cup (145 g) blueberries for 1 cup (166 g) strawberries. Arrange 1 cup (145 g) blueberries over cream cheese in pie crust; spoon half the gelatin mixture over berries; top with 1 cup sliced strawberries and spoon remaining gelatin mixture over.

Strawberry–Banana Pie—Make recipe as above, substituting sugar-free strawberry-banana gelatin for the strawberry gelatin and 1 small sliced banana for 1 cup (166 g) strawberries. Arrange banana over cream cheese; spoon half the gelatin mixture over; top with 1 cup (166 g) sliced strawberries and spoon remaining gelatin mixture over.

Per Serving: **Calories: 165; % of calories from fat: 38; Fat (g): 6.9; Saturated fat (g): 1.6; Cholesterol (mg): 2.3; Sodium (mg): 330; Protein (g): 8.9; Carbohydrate (g): 17.1** Exchanges: **Milk: 0.0; Vegetable: 0.0; Fruit: 0.0; Bread: 1.0; Meat: 1.0; Fat: 1.0**

CHOCOLATE YOGURT PIE

This pie is quick and easy to assemble, especially if you purchase a crust and reduced-fat brownies. This recipe comes from Diabetes Snacks, Treats, and Easy Eats *by Barbara Grunes.*

8 SERVINGS (1 SLICE PER SERVING)

> 1 (9-inch [22.5-cm]) Graham Cracker Crust (see recipe on page 133)
> 3½ cups (826 mL) plain low-fat yogurt
> 1 packet (½ ounce [14 g]) sugar-free hot cocoa mix
> 6 reduced-fat brownies, crumbled, store-bought or home-made (see recipe on page 126)

1. Refrigerate the crust for at least 20 minutes.

2. Mix the yogurt with cocoa mix in a large bowl. Measure 2 cups of the crumbled brownies and fold into the yogurt mixture. Mound the filling into the crust. Cover the pie lightly with foil.

3. Freeze the pie until firm, 2 hours.

4. Just before serving, remove the pie from the freezer and let stand at room temperature to soften slightly. Cut into 8 slices.

Per Serving: **Calories:** 221; **% calories from fat:** 35; **Fat (g):** 8.5; **Saturated fat (g):** 2.5; **Cholesterol (mg):** 22.7; **Sodium (mg):** 343; **Protein (g):** 8.8; **Carbohydrate (g):** 26.8 Exchanges: **Milk:** 0.0; **Vegetable:** 0.0; **Fruit:** 0.0; **Bread:** 2.0; **Meat:** 0.0; **Fat:** 1.5

LEMON PIE

For a change of pace, make the crust with gingersnaps instead of graham crackers. The easiest way to make graham cracker or gingersnap crumbs is in the food processor or blender.

8 SERVINGS

> 1 Graham Cracker Crust (recipe follows)
> 1 (0.32-ounce [8 g]) package sugar-free lemon flavored gelatin
> ¼ cup (59 mL) boiling water
> 2 (6-ounce [170-g]) containers lemon pie-flavored light yogurt
> 1 container (8 ounces [224 g]) frozen fat-free whipped topping

1. In a large bowl dissolve gelatin in ¼ cup (59 mL) boiling water. Cool until syrupy. Stir in yogurt and fold in whipped topping.

2. Spoon the mixture into the prepared crust. Refrigerate for 2 to 4 hours or overnight.

3. When ready to serve, remove from the refrigerator and cut into 8 equal servings.

GRAHAM CRACKER CRUST

1 (9-INCH [22.5-CM]) PIE CRUST TO SERVE 8

      5 tablespoons (70 g) reduced-calorie margarine, melted
      1¼ cups (125 g) graham cracker crumbs
      ½ teaspoon (2.5 mL) ground cinnamon

1. Preheat oven to 350°F (180°C). Stir the margarine, crumbs, and cinnamon together in a bowl. Press the mixture firmly into the bottom and up the sides of a 9-inch (22.5-cm) pie pan.

2. Bake 10 minutes. Cool on wire rack. Cut into 8 slices.

Per Serving: **Calories: 167; % calories from fat: 40; Fat (g): 7.4; Saturated fat (g): 4.1; Cholesterol (mg): 0.63; Sodium (mg): 230; Protein (g): 3.4; Carbohydrate (g): 21.8** Exchanges: **Milk: 0.0; Vegetable: 0.0; Fruit: 0.0; Bread: 1.5; Meat: 0.0; Fat: 1.5**

BISCOTTI

For a more intense flavor, add 1 teaspoon anise flavoring and 2 table-spoons grated lemon zest to the dough.

22 SLICES (1 SLICE PER SERVING)

Butter-flavored cooking spray
2 cups (242 g) all-purpose flour
⅓ cup (67 g) sugar
2 tablespoons (30 mL) anise seeds or poppy seeds
1 teaspoon (5 mL) baking powder
½ teaspoon (2.5 mL) baking soda
1 cup (236 mL) egg substitute

1. Position a rack in the center of the oven and preheat oven to 325°F (165°C). Lightly coat a nonstick baking sheet with cooking spray.

2. Combine the flour, sugar, anise seeds, baking powder, baking soda, and egg substitute in a bowl using electric mixer.

3. Knead the dough with clean, damp hands until it holds together. Add a little more flour, if necessary, during kneading to keep the dough from sticking.

4. Shape the dough into a log almost the length of the prepared baking sheet. Lightly coat the top of the log with cooking spray.

5. Bake until log becomes firm to the touch, 35 minutes. Remove from oven and cool slightly on baking sheet. While log is still warm, cut diagonally into scant ½-inch (13-mm) thick slices.

6. Lay slices cut side down on baking sheet. Bake another 15 minutes or until biscotti are crisp. Cool completely on wire racks. Store in an airtight container in a cool, dry place.

Per Serving: **Calories: 60; % calories from fat: 3; Fat (g): 0; Saturated fat (g): 0;** **Cholesterol (mg): 0; Sodium (mg): 69; Protein (g): 2.4; Carbohydrate (g): 12.1** Exchanges: **Milk: 0.0; Vegetable: 0.0; Fruit: 0.0; Bread: 1.0; Meat: 0.0; Fat: 0.0**

ORANGE MERINGUE COOKIES

Meringues bake better on a dry day. For optimum volume, use fresh eggs that have stood on the counter until they are at room temperature. To quickly warm eggs, place them in a bowl of tepid water.

ABOUT 18 COOKIES (1 COOKIE PER SERVING)

> **Vegetable oil cooking spray**
> **2 egg whites, at room temperature**
> **⅓ cup (67 g) sugar**
> **1 teaspoon (5 mL) each: cream of tartar, orange extract**

1. Preheat oven to 275°F (140°C). Lightly coat a baking sheet with cooking spray. Line the sprayed sheet with foil or parchment baking paper.

2. Beat the egg whites with an electric mixer until soft peaks form. Sprinkle the egg whites with the sugar and cream of tartar. Continue beating until stiff peaks form. Add the orange extract and fold in gently by hand with a rubber spatula.

3. Drop the egg white mixture by the tablespoonful onto the baking sheet.

4. Bake 45 minutes. Turn the oven off and cool the cookies in the oven with the oven door closed. The cookies should be firm to the touch. Store the cookies in an airtight container.

Per Serving: **Calories: 17; % calories from fat: 0; Fat (g): 0; Saturated fat (g): 0; Cholesterol (mg): 0; Sodium (mg): 6; Protein (g): 0.4; Carbohydrate (g): 3.7** Exchanges: **Milk: 0.0; Vegetable: 0.0; Fruit: 0.0; Bread: 0.25; Meat: 0.0; Fat: 0.0**

CHOCOLATE CHIP COOKIES

America's favorite cookie—best eaten warm!

5 DOZEN COOKIES (1 EACH)

> 2½ cups (303 g) all-purpose flour
> ½ teaspoon (2.5 mL) each: baking soda, salt
> 8 tablespoons (114 g) margarine or butter, room temperature
> 1 cup (225 g) packed light brown sugar
> ½ cup (100 g) granulated sugar
> 1 egg
> 1 teaspoon (5 mL) vanilla
> ⅓ cup (79 mL) fat-free milk
> ½ package (12-ounce [340-g] size) reduced-fat semisweet chocolate morsels

1. Preheat oven to 375°F (190°C). Grease cookie sheets.

2. Combine the flour, baking soda, and salt.

3. Beat the margarine and sugars in a medium bowl until fluffy; beat in egg and vanilla. Mix in the flour mixture alternately with milk, beginning and ending with the dry ingredients. Mix in chocolate morsels. Drop dough by tablespoonfuls onto prepared cookie sheets. Bake until browned, about 10 minutes. Cool on wire racks.

Per Serving: **Calories:** 66; **% of calories from fat:** 27; **Fat (g):** 2; **Saturated fat (g):** 0.7; **Cholesterol (mg):** 3.6; **Sodium (mg):** 70; **Protein (g):** 0.8; **Carbohydrate (g):** 11.2 Exchanges: **Milk:** 0.0; **Vegetable:** 0.0; **Fruit:** 0.0; **Bread:** 0.5; **Meat:** 0.0; **Fat:** 0.5

SOFT MOLASSES COOKIES

Fill your home with the scent of spices when you bake these cookies.

3 DOZEN COOKIES (1 EACH)

> 1¼ cups (151 g) all-purpose flour
> 2 teaspoons (10 mL) baking soda
> ½ teaspoon (2.5 mL) each: ground cinnamon, ginger
> ¼ teaspoon (1.25 mL) each: ground nutmeg, salt
> ¼ cup (48 g) vegetable shortening
> ½ cup (113 g) packed dark brown sugar
> 1 egg yolk
> ¼ cup (59 mL) light molasses
> 2 tablespoons (30 mL) water
> ½ cup (83 g) currants or chopped raisins

1. Preheat oven to 350°F (180°C). Grease cookie sheets.

2. Combine the flour, baking soda, cinnamon, ginger, nutmeg, and salt.

3. Beat the shortening, brown sugar, and egg yolk in a medium bowl until blended. Mix in the flour mixture, alternately with combined molasses and water, beginning and ending with dry ingredients. Mix in the currants. Drop mixture by rounded teaspoons onto prepared cookie sheets. Bake until lightly browned (cookies will be soft), 8 to 10 minutes. Cool on wire racks.

Per Serving: **Calories:** 53; **% of calories from fat:** 25; **Fat (g):** 1.5; **Saturated fat (g):** 0.4; **Cholesterol (mg):** 5.9; **Sodium (mg):** 89; **Protein (g):** 0.6; **Carbohydrate (g):** 9.3 Exchanges: **Milk:** 0.0; **Vegetable:** 0.0; **Fruit:** 0.0; **Bread:** 0.5; **Meat:** 0.0; **Fat:** 0.0

TART LEMON DAINTIES

Enjoy the subtle lemon flavor of these tiny crisp cookies—perfect with coffee or tea.

4 DOZEN COOKIES (1 EACH)

2 cups (242 g) all-purpose flour
1 teaspoon (5 mL) baking powder
¼ teaspoon (1.25 mL) salt
4 tablespoons (57 g) margarine or butter, room temperature
1 cup (200 g) granulated sugar
1 egg
3 tablespoons (45 mL) fat-free milk
2 teaspoons (10 mL) lemon juice
1 teaspoon (5 mL) grated lemon zest

1. Combine the flour, baking powder, and salt.

2. Beat the margarine, sugar, egg, milk, lemon juice, and lemon zest in bowl until blended. Mix in the flour mixture. Refrigerate until chilled, 2 to 3 hours.

3. Preheat oven to 375°F (190°C). Grease cookie sheets.

4. Roll half of the dough on a floured surface to ¼-inch (6-mm) thickness; cut into rounds or decorative shapes with 1½-inch (4-cm) cutter. Repeat with the remaining dough. Bake on prepared cookie sheets until lightly browned, 7 to 8 minutes. Cool on wire racks.

Per Serving: **Calories: 46;** % of calories from fat: 22; **Fat (g): 1.1;** Saturated fat (g): 0.2; **Cholesterol (mg): 4.4;** Sodium (mg): 35; **Protein (g): 0.7;** Carbohydrate (g): 8.2 Exchanges: **Milk: 0.0;** Vegetable: 0.0; **Fruit: 0.0;** Bread: 0.5; **Meat: 0.0;** Fat: 0.0

GRANOLA LACE COOKIES

When the cookies are still warm, they can be rolled or folded over the handle of a wooden spoon, or "pinched" in the center to form bow shapes. Bake only 4 to 6 cookies at a time, as they must be handled quickly and carefully before cooling.

4 DOZEN COOKIES (1 EACH)

> 4 tablespoons (57 g) margarine or butter, room temperature
> ¼ cup each: granulated sugar (50 g), packed light brown sugar (56 g)
> 2 egg whites
> 1 tablespoon (15 mL) orange juice
> ¼–½ teaspoon (1.25–2.5 mL) orange extract
> ½ cup each: finely crushed reduced-fat granola without raisins (55 g), all-purpose flour (61 g)
> ¼ teaspoon (1.25 mL) each: baking soda, salt
> 2 teaspoons (10 mL) grated orange zest

1. Preheat oven to 400°F (200°C). Line cookie sheets with parchment paper.

2. Beat all ingredients in a large bowl until smooth. Drop rounded ½ teaspoons (2.5 mL) dough 3 inches (7.5 cm) apart on prepared cookie sheets, making 4 to 6 cookies per pan. Bake until lightly browned, about 3 minutes. Let stand until firm enough to remove from pans, about 1 minute. Cool on wire racks.

Per Serving: **Calories: 27; % of calories from fat: 33; Fat (g): 1; Saturated fat (g): 0.2; Cholesterol (mg): 0; Sodium (mg): 35; Protein (g): 0.4; Carbohydrate (g): 4.1** Exchanges: **Milk: 0.0; Vegetable: 0.0; Fruit: 0.0; Bread: 0.5; Meat: 0.0; Fat: 0.0**

RASPBERRY-ALMOND BARS

A pretty bar cookie with a rich-tasting shortbread pastry.

2 DOZEN COOKIES (1 EACH)

> 2 cups (242 g) all-purpose flour
> 3½ teaspoons (13 g) Equal® for Recipes or 12 packets Equal® sweetener
> ⅛ teaspoon (.625 mL) salt
> 8 tablespoons (114 g) cold margarine or butter, cut into pieces
> 1 large egg, beaten
> 1 tablespoon (15 mL) fat-free milk or water
> ⅔ cup (214 g) seedless raspberry preserves
> 1 teaspoon (10 mL) cornstarch
> ¼–⅓ cup (27–36 g) finely chopped almonds, walnuts or pecans, toasted

1. Preheat oven to 400°F (200°C). Grease an 11 × 7-inch (28 × 18-cm) baking dish.

2. Combine the flour, Equal® for Recipes, and salt in a medium bowl; cut in the margarine until mixture resembles coarse crumbs. Mix in the egg and milk. Press mixture evenly in bottom of prepared baking dish. Bake until edges of crust are browned, about 15 minutes. Cool on a wire rack.

3. Mix the preserves and cornstarch in a small saucepan; heat to boiling, stirring until thickened, about 1 minute; cool 5 minutes. Spread mixture over cooled crust; sprinkle with almonds. Bake until preserves are thick and bubbly, about 15 minutes. Cool on a wire rack.

Per Serving: **Calories:** 96; **% of calories from fat:** 45; **Fat (g):** 4.6; **Saturated fat (g):** 0.9; **Cholesterol (mg):** 8.8; **Sodium (mg):** 69; **Protein (g):** 2.1; **Carbohydrate (g):** 10.5 Exchanges: **Milk:** 0.0; **Vegetable:** 0.0; **Fruit:** 0.0; **Bread:** 0.5; **Meat:** 0.0; **Fat:** 1.0

BANANA–CHOCOLATE SHERBET

Bananas contain fiber, potassium, and other healthful nutrients that make them a good food choice, although in moderation because of their relatively high carbohydrate content. Puréed bananas create a smooth, creamy consistency, almost like ice cream.

6 SERVINGS

> 5 ripe bananas, peeled and cut into chunks
> 2 tablespoons (30 mL) cocoa powder
> 1 packet sugar substitute

1. Purée the bananas with the cocoa powder and sugar substitute in a food processor or blender. Spoon the mixture into a covered container and freeze for 2 hours or until firm.

2. When ready to serve, scoop the sherbet into footed glasses. Serve immediately.

Per Serving: **Calories:** 95; **% calories from fat:** 6; **Fat (g):** 0.7; **Saturated fat (g):** 0.3; **Cholesterol (mg):** 0; **Sodium (mg):** 1; **Protein (g):** 1.3; **Carbohydrate (g):** 24.2 Exchanges: **Milk:** 0.0; **Vegetable:** 0.0; **Fruit:** 1.5; **Bread:** 0.0; **Meat:** 0.0; **Fat:** 0.0

PUMPKIN CHEESECAKE >

A creamy smooth cheesecake, scented with holiday flavors of pumpkin and spices.

12 TO 14 SERVINGS

¾ cup each: ground reduced-fat graham crackers (75 g) and gingersnap cookies (75 g), divided

8¼ teaspoons (30 g) Equal® for Recipes or 27 packets Equal® sweetener, divided

4–5 tablespoons (57–71 g) margarine or butter, melted

16 ounces (454 g) fat-free cream cheese, room temperature

8 ounces (224 g) reduced-fat cream cheese, room temperature

1 cup (245 g) canned pumpkin

3 eggs

2 teaspoons (10 mL) ground cinnamon

1 teaspoon (5 mL) each: ground cloves, ginger

2 tablespoons (30 mL) cornstarch

1 cup (236 mL) light whipped topping

Chopped toasted pecans, for garnish

1. Preheat oven to 350°F (180°C).

2. Mix the graham cracker and gingersnap crumbs, 1 teaspoon (5 mL) Equal® for Recipes, and margarine in bottom of a 9-inch (22.5-cm) springform pan; reserve 2 tablespoons (30 mL) crumb mixture. Pat the remaining mixture evenly on bottom and ½ inch up side of pan. Bake until lightly browned, about 8 minutes. Cool on a wire rack. Reduce oven temperature to 300°F (150°C).

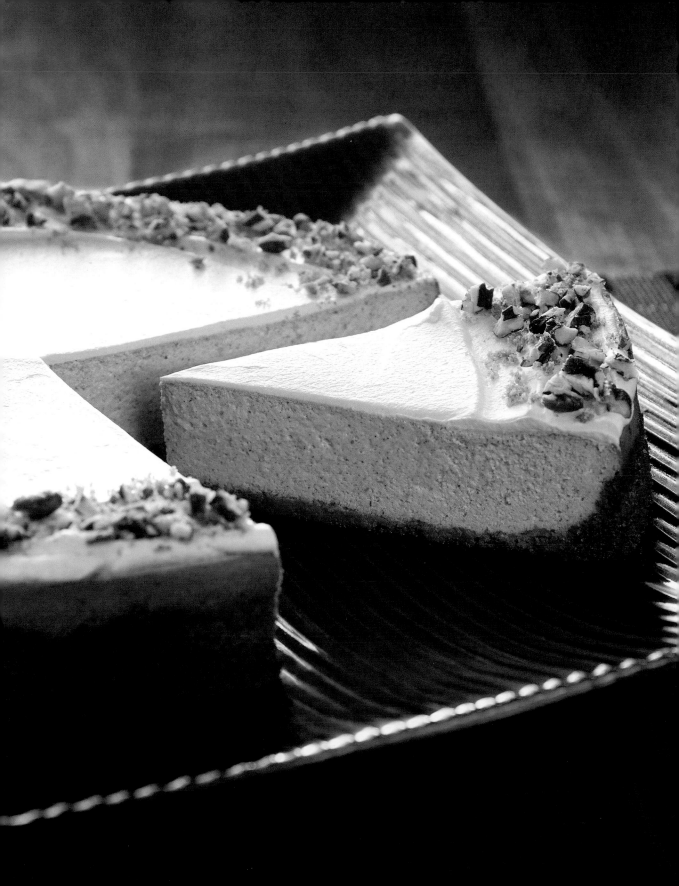

3. Beat the cream cheese and remaining 7¼ teaspoons (36.25 mL) Equal® for Recipes until smooth in a large bowl; beat in the remaining ingredients, except whipped topping and pecans. Pour over crust in springform pan.

4. Bake at 300°F (150°C) just until set in the center, 45 to 60 minutes. Turn the oven off and let the cheesecake cool in oven with door ajar for 3 hours. Refrigerate 8 hours or overnight.

5. Remove the side of the springform pan; place cheesecake on a serving plate. Spread with light whipped topping and reserved crumb mixture. Sprinkle with pecans.

Per Serving: **Calories: 213**; % of calories from fat: **42**; Fat (g): **9.8**; Saturated fat (g): **4.3**; Cholesterol (mg): **47.2**; Sodium (mg): **444**; Protein (g): **12.1**; Carbohydrate (g): **18.2** Exchanges: Milk: **0.0**; Vegetable: **0.0**; Fruit: **0.0**; Bread: **1.0**; Meat: **1.0**; Fat: **2.0**

CHEESECAKE CUPCAKES

No need to frost, as these chocolate cupcakes are baked with a topping of cream cheese.

20 SERVINGS (1 EACH)

¾ cup each: all-purpose flour (91 g), sugar (150 g), reduced-fat buttermilk (178 mL)
⅓ cup (29 g) unsweetened cocoa
¾ teaspoon (3.75 mL) baking soda
½ teaspoon (2.5 mL) salt
¼ cup (48 g) shortening
1 egg
1 teaspoon (5 mL) vanilla
Cheesecake Topping (recipe follows)
½ cup (90 g) reduced-fat semisweet chocolate morsels

1. Preheat oven to 350°F (180°C). Line 20 muffin cups with paper liners.

2. Combine all ingredients, except the Cheesecake Topping and chocolate morsels, in a large bowl. Beat at low speed until blended; beat at high speed 3 minutes, scraping side of bowl occasionally. Pour batter into prepared muffin cups, filling each about half full.

3. Spread about 1 tablespoon (15 mL) Cheesecake Topping over batter in each, covering completely. Sprinkle each with about 1 teaspoon chocolate morsels. Bake until golden, about 30 minutes. Cool in pans on wire rack.

CHEESECAKE TOPPING

> 8 ounces (227 g) fat-free cream cheese, room temperature
> ½ cup (100 g) sugar
> 1 egg

1. Mix all ingredients until smooth.

Per Serving: **Calories: 136**; **% of calories from fat: 29**; **Fat (g): 4.6**; **Saturated fat (g): 2.3**; **Cholesterol (mg): 22.5**; **Sodium (mg): 186**; **Protein (g): 3.4**; **Carbohydrate (g): 21.7** Exchanges: **Milk: 0.0**; **Vegetable: 0.0**; **Fruit: 0.0**; **Bread: 1.5**; **Meat: 0.0**; **Fat: 0.5**

OLD-FASHIONED APPLE CRISP

Juicy apples baked with a crisp sweet-spiced topping will warm hearts in any season.

3½ teaspoons (13 g) Equal® for Recipes or 12 packets
   Equal® sweetener
1 tablespoon (15 mL) cornstarch
¾ cup (59 mL) unsweetened apple juice
1 teaspoon (5 mL) grated lemon zest
4 cups (440 g) sliced peeled apples
Crispy Spiced Topping (recipe follows)

1. Preheat oven to 400°F (200°C).

2. Combine Equal® for Recipes, cornstarch, apple juice, and lemon zest in a medium saucepan; heat over medium-high heat to boiling, whisking until thickened, about 1 minute. Add the apples and simmer, uncovered, until the apples begin to lose their crispness, about 5 minutes.

3. Transfer the mixture to an 8-inch (20-cm) square baking pan; sprinkle with Crispy Spiced Topping. Bake until topping is browned and apples are tender, about 25 minutes. Serve warm.

CRISPY SPICED TOPPING

MAKES ABOUT ¾ CUP (177 ML)

> ¼ cup (30 g) all-purpose flour
>
> 2½ teaspoons (9 g) Equal® for Recipes or 8 packets Equal® sweetener
>
> 1 teaspoon (5 mL) ground cinnamon
>
> ½ teaspoon (2.5 mL) ground nutmeg
>
> 4 tablespoons (57 g) cold margarine or butter, cut into pieces
>
> ¼ cup each: quick-cooking oats (23 g), flaked coconut (23 g)

1. Combine the flour, Equal® for Recipes, cinnamon, and nutmeg in a small bowl; cut in the margarine until mixture resembles coarse crumbs. Stir in the oats and coconut.

Per Serving: **Calories:** 198; **% of calories from fat:** 41; **Fat (g):** 9.3; **Saturated fat (g):** 2.5; **Cholesterol (mg):** 0; **Sodium (mg):** 93; **Protein (g):** 4.8; **Carbohydrate (g):** 25.7
Exchanges: **Milk:** 0.0; **Vegetable:** 0.0; **Fruit:** 1.0; **Bread:** 1.5; **Meat:** 0.0; **Fat:** 2.0

BAKED CUSTARD WITH ORANGE SAUCE

This delicate custard is complemented with a sweet orange sauce.

6 SERVINGS (ABOUT 2/3 CUP [158 ML] EACH)

> 1 quart (0.95 L) fat-free milk
>
> 5 eggs, lightly beaten
>
> 5 teaspoons (18 g) Equal® for Recipes or 16 packets Equal® sweetener
>
> 2 teaspoons (10 mL) vanilla
>
> Orange Sauce (recipe follows)

1. Preheat oven to 325°F (165°C).

2. Heat the milk just to simmering in a medium saucepan. Mix the eggs, milk, Equal® for Recipes, and vanilla. Pour mixture through strainer into an ungreased 1-quart (948-mL) casserole or soufflé dish.

3. Place the casserole in roasting pan on center oven rack; pour 2 inches (5 cm) hot water into pan. Bake, covered, until custard is set and a sharp knife inserted halfway between center and edge comes out clean, 1 to 1¼ hours. Remove the casserole from the roasting pan; cool to room temperature on a wire rack. Refrigerate until chilled; serve with Orange Sauce.

ORANGE SAUCE

ABOUT 1¾ CUPS (415 ML)

¾ **cup (177 mL) orange juice**

1 tablespoon (15 mL) cornstarch

1 teaspoon (5 mL) Equal® for Recipes or 3 packets Equal® sweetener

1 cup (180 g) orange segments

1. Mix the orange juice and cornstarch in a small saucepan; heat to boiling, whisking until thickened, 2 to 3 minutes. Stir in Equal® for Recipes and orange segments. Cool to room temperature; refrigerate until chilled.

VARIATION

Baked Chocolate Custard—Make recipe as above, increasing Equal® for Recipes to 6¼ teaspoons (23 g) and adding ⅓ cup (29 g) Dutch process cocoa to the milk mixture. Serve with dollops of light whipped topping.

Per Serving: **Calories: 174**; % of calories from fat: **24**; Fat (g): **4.6**; Saturated fat (g): **1.5**; Cholesterol (mg): **179.6**; Sodium (mg): **138**; Protein (g): **14.3**; Carbohydrate (g): **17.7** Exchanges: **Milk: 1.0**; **Vegetable: 0.0**; **Fruit: 0.0**; **Bread: 0.5**; **Meat: 1.0**; **Fat: 0.0**

INDEX

Also from Agate Surrey

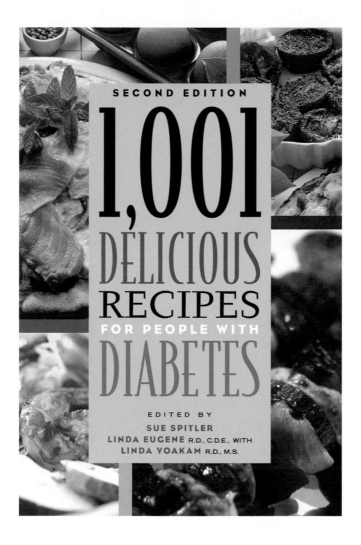

SURREY
BOOKS

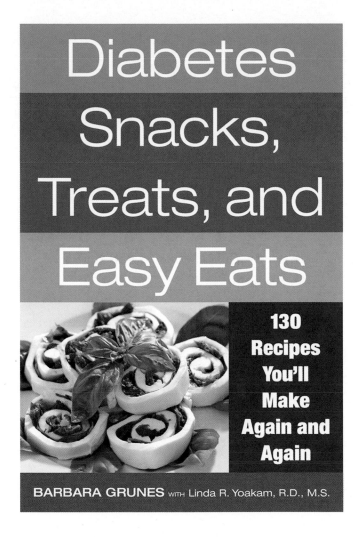

ABOUT THE SERIES

Each of the books in the *101* series feature delicious, diverse, and accessible recipes—101 of them, to be exact. Scattered throughout each book are beautiful full-color photographs to show you just what the dish should look like. The *101* series books also feature a simple, contemporary design that's as practical as it is elegant, with measures calculated in both traditional and metric quantities.

ABOUT THE EDITOR

Perrin Davis is co-editor of Surrey's *101* series. She lives with her family in suburban Chicago.